# woman
## *to* *woman*

A Handbook for Women
Newly Diagnosed with
Breast Cancer

# woman
## *to woman*

Hester Hill Schnipper, LICSW
Joan Feinberg Berns, Ph.D.

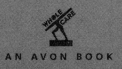

AN AVON BOOK

AVON BOOKS, INC.
1350 Avenue of the Americas
New York, New York 10019

Copyright © 1996, 1999 by Hester Hill Schnipper, LICSW and
Joan Feinberg Berns, Ph.D.
Front cover design by Thomson Financial
Interior design by Pauline Neuwirth, Neuwirth & Associates, Inc.
Published by arrangement with the authors
ISBN: 0-380-80632-0
www.avonbooks.com/wholecare

Library of Congress Cataloging in Publication Data:

Schnipper, Hester Hill
    Woman to woman : a handbook for women newly diagnosed with
    breast cancer / Hester Hill Schnipper, Joan Feinberg Berns.
        p.   cm.
    "An Avon book."
    Includes bibliographical references and index.
    1. Breast Cancer—Popular works.    I. Berns, Joan Feinberg.
    II. Title.
RC280.B8B475   1999                                    99-29595
616.99'449—dc21                                           CIP

First WholeCare Printing: October 1999

WHOLECARE TRADEMARK REG. U.S. PAT. OFF. AND IN OTHER COUNTRIES,
MARCA REGISTRADA, HECHO EN U.S.A.

Printed in the U.S.A.

OPM 10 9 8 7 6 5 4 3 2 1

We dedicate this book to our husbands, Steven Berns
and Lowell Schnipper, and to our children,
who are our future:

David, Sarah, and Andrew Berns; Katharine and Julia Hill

# acknowledgments

We wish to express our gratitude to the many people who advised, supported, and encouraged us along the way.

Several members of the Beth Israel Hospital took the time to read and comment on our manuscript at different stages of its evolution. We owe special thanks to one surgeon for his interest and support from the very beginning. Dr. Clinton Koufman not only gave his time and attention to our project, he also provided seed money for the original handbook from the Joseph Koufman Memorial Fund.

We are very grateful to Dr. Lowell Schnipper who, for both personal and professional reasons, carefully read every word of this manuscript, and to Steven Berns, who spent innumerable hours helping us with many aspects of this project.

Cathie Ragovi, M.D., read through our typescript and responded with her enthusiastic support and encouragement.

We also want to thank publicly the many hundreds of women we have met face-to-face who, like the two of us, are also living with breast cancer each day and night. We are grateful for their generosity in sharing their personal stories and their wisdom with us. Special appreciation to Jane Hyman for her steadfast belief in the importance of our project.

To our homegrown and best support team—our families—whose love has kept us alive in more ways than we can express here, we offer our most profound and abundant gratitude.

# to the reader

The first version of this book was prepared by the authors for use by and within the Beth Israel Deaconess Medical Center in Boston, Massachusetts. In this revised and expanded book, the authors continue to make every attempt to portray the diagnosis and treatment of breast cancer as accurately as possible. However, since they are not physicians, the authors and the publisher strongly recommend that you speak with your specialists in the event that this book conflicts with any information you have obtained elsewhere or if you feel uncomfortable or unsure about any of its subject matter.

You are encouraged to use original printed copies of this book for any noncommercial, personal purpose whatsoever. However, since this is a copyrighted work, we ask that you not make any copies of the complete book or any portions thereof without the express prior written authorization of the publishers.

This book is not an official publication of any organization or company and does not represent the authoritative views of any physician or employee of any hospital or organization. It has been written by two women from their own experiences and comes from the heart as friendly advice intended to help others as they confront a new diagnosis of breast cancer. The Beth Israel Deaconess Medical Center of Boston, Massachusetts, Avon Books, and the authors expressly disclaim all liability with respect to the book's subject matter or its use.

# contents

CHAPTER ONE

*introduction*

Even though you may have heard the statistics, known that one in eight American women will hear those words at some point in her lifetime, you probably never thought it would be you. The odds are good that you do not have a family history of this illness. You may well have always taken good enough care of yourself, paid attention to your diet and to exercise, and thought you were in excellent health. The truth is that although your overall good health will help you get through these next months, you cannot protect yourself from developing this disease. You did not develop breast cancer because of anything you did or did not do. This did not happen to you because in some way you did not take good enough care of yourself. It is not because of where you live, what you eat, the wine you might enjoy occasionally, the exercise you did not do, or the stress of your job or family life. Breast cancer just happens. It is the result of a series of complex biological events that *you could not control*. No one yet understands what triggers the abnormal cell growth that becomes cancer. But you are not responsible!

We will remind you of this again, but it is so important that it bears repeating. *Breast cancer is not a medical emergency*. You have some time to consider your options and to make careful decisions.

We believe that we can help you. The two of us who wrote this book envision sharing with you what you would hear if you could at this moment sit with ten women who have been through this nightmare. Most important, each of us brings her own personal experience of being a woman with breast cancer. Hester has been an oncology social worker, working with women living with breast cancer, for more than twenty years. Joan, who is a professional writer with a doctorate in English and American literature, works in major gifts fund-raising at Brandeis University in Massachusetts; she came to one of Hester's support groups, and the idea for this book grew from that association.

You might want to know how this book came to be. A year after we were diagnosed and treated, we both felt very grateful for having passed through the first round of our personal encounter with this disease. Both of us wanted to do something concrete to help other women just beginning their struggle with breast cancer. We discussed what form this impulse might take and decided that a simple handbook of thoughts and advice might be valuable and useful to other women and their family and friends.

Over a few months in the fall of 1994 we stapled together sheets of paper with tips and advice, and we left these pages out in the Hematology/Oncology Division of our hospital. They disappeared rapidly. We wondered if we could get help producing a small handbook. A year later, with help from a group of young women who were talented graphic designers in the Communications Division at Thomson Financial Services in Boston and with support from the Beth Israel Hospital in Boston, we had 5,000 copies of our handbook printed for us at cost courtesy of R. R. Donnelley through the kind advocacy of Marilyn Brady. The handbook, *Woman to Woman: Thoughts and Advice for Women Newly Diagnosed with Breast Cancer*, appeared in February 1996 and was made available to patients through their surgeons, medical oncologists, and radiation oncologists at the Beth Israel Hospital in Boston.

Over the following year, the handbook was also distributed through several other Boston area hospitals as well as through doctors' offices, hospitals, and clinics around the country. Because of our handbook's popularity, the hospital (now known as Beth Israel Deaconess Medical Center) asked us to reprint it, and in the spring of 1998, a second run of 15,000 copies was produced. One copy was read by a patient who found it so helpful that she brought it to the attention of a friend at Avon Books in New York City. From January 1998 to May 1999, Hester and Joan worked with their editor, Ann McKay Thoroman, at Avon Books to produce the book you are now holding.

You may also be wondering who we are personally. We are both daughters, siblings, wives, and mothers. Between us we have six children ranging in age from eighteen to twenty-eight, and a hundred years of life experience. At the time of our treatments six years ago, we each had a preadolescent child of twelve.

We talked about this book with hundreds of other women

and feel privileged to have the opportunity to pass on the cumulative wisdom of so many to you, our readers. Each of us who contributed to this project, either directly or indirectly, has received the same diagnosis; we have stood where you are now standing; we know you feel (or will feel) many strong emotions, including fear, anxiety, bewilderment, denial, depression, and/or anger. "Why me?" you may ask, or at least, "Why me at this point in my life?" This book aims to share with you the kind of tips and advice we wish we had heard after diagnosis and before treatment.

You may want to respond, as many of us have at various times, "I'm too young/busy/healthy to have cancer!" None of us felt we had time for a serious disease, and frankly, none of us wanted to deal with cancer. But each of us has found ways to cope with this new and unwelcome predicament, just as you will. An excellent way to begin is to talk to other women with breast cancer, particularly those who have had treatments similar to the ones recommended for you. You will find, as we have, that no one understands how you feel as clearly as someone who has been through the same crisis; other women living with breast cancer will provide a sympathetic ear, a mirror for your emotions, and a host of practical tips.

## Finding Support: Peer Groups and Professional Facilitators

WE CANNOT OVEREMPHASIZE THE IMPORTANCE OF MAKING A CONNECTION WITH ANOTHER WOMAN WHO HAS LIVED THROUGH BREAST CANCER. She will help you in many, many ways—more ways than we can begin to enumerate here. FIND HER.

What we are about to say now will probably seem crazy to you right now, but someday you too will recognize that there has been a silver lining to this experience. Most of us truly believe that the most precious benefit of this entire ordeal is the relationships we have developed with the other women whom we have met. The community of women who have had breast cancer is enormous and remarkable. You now have friends, sisters beyond number, and each is waiting to help in any way she can. We mean it sincerely when we tell each other "Call me anytime."

You have been through a lot already; you have found the strength you needed to confront difficult moments: mammograms, biopsies, X-rays, bone scans, and blood tests, and certainly the phone call from hell. You may feel devastated; you feel you can't deal with one more decision; you may feel as though you want to snuggle under the covers and sleep so that you won't have to address all the overwhelming questions that crowd into your mind. This is all normal and common. Of course you know that you will have to make decisions and choices; remember that it is okay not to like any of this. No one would choose to be in this predicament; none of us voluntarily made that choice, either. We are all reluctant, if not rebellious, members of a sorority we never wanted to join.

As you have already discovered, the time around the initial diagnosis is very difficult, painful, and stressful. You should know that you are at a very bad time emotionally; you may have heard from your doctors that this is the very worst time. Believe it. Once you have made the necessary decisions and once you have begun treatment, you will feel more settled, more in control. We are not suggesting that you will feel happy or carefree, not at all. But we are suggesting that you will experience some measure of relief. Before you arrive at this point, you will need to do your homework. It is *very important* that you make informed decisions about your treatment. Remember, it is *your* body and it is *your* life.

These first days are harder than anything yet to come. We know you don't believe this now, but you will look back and see that this is true. Right now, however, it is normal to feel that your life is over, that your life is out of control, and even, perhaps, that you are crazy. Many women report, during the inevitable sleepless nights, that they are lying awake planning their funerals. Some of us stop eating. Some of us eat continuously. Most of us cry a lot. You will be impatient and short-tempered. You may either tell everyone you meet about your diagnosis, including the cashier in the market and the UPS deliveryman, or you may tell almost no one.

One woman remembers getting out of her car in a crowded parking lot to scream at another driver who had just outmaneuvered her. Another tells of breaking down at an airport when her flight was delayed. Many normally patient mothers yell at their children and then feel especially guilty, since they are simultaneously terrified of leaving these same children motherless.

Try to be easy on yourself. Lower your usual expectations. During this initial diagnostic phase, it is probably wise to cancel what you can. Delegate. Reschedule. Focus on yourself and your own needs. Some women find it really helpful to get away for a day or two. Others find it difficult to be alone and ask friends and family to be with them. This is the time to put yourself first and to ask for help, as you need it.

*Breast cancer is not a medical emergency. It is a crisis in your life, but it is not an emergency.* You can safely take some time to seek another opinion. You need to know what your choices are. After your doctor has explained to you what alternatives would be reasonable for you, you should prepare yourself to make as fully informed a decision as you can. There are many sources of information: books, pamphlets, journal and magazine articles, the Internet, the National Cancer Institute and American Cancer Society information hotlines, etc. (see the resources section for further information). Take the time you need to gather information from different sources. Contact other women who have had breast cancer treatment; talk to them about their experiences and ask questions. Many of us have called friends of friends, perfect strangers, who have had breast cancer. Invariably, we found these women were supportive and helpful in answering our questions. Depend on the kindness of strangers. As you gather information, you may find numbers or statistics that are disturbing or frightening. Ask your doctor for clarification, and remember that you are an individual, not a statistic! That is, a statistic is not your personal fate, but is a general observation about a large number of women.

Many women find it helpful to read about breast cancer and treatment choices; many women also seek out written accounts of others' personal experience. *Remember as you read that all specific medical information, including statistics, is out of date by the time you read it.* Both treatments for breast cancer and scientific understanding of the illness are changing constantly. If you want to read the most current medical journal articles, ask one of your doctors for references. If you prefer to read nothing, that is fine, too. Don't let other people force their coping styles on you. Most women find that at some point during this process, they have read enough; they reach a saturation point. Friends will likely continue to send you articles or books; feel free to decide not to read them. Feel free, also, to tell well-meaning friends and family members to stop sending you these articles if you are upset by receiving them. At the end of this book there is a bibliography and a resources section we hope you will find useful.

Many women with breast cancer find it helpful to talk with a therapist about their concerns. Your friends and family may not be able to provide all of the support you need, and a therapist who is knowledgeable about cancer and cancer treatment can be an invaluable resource. It is really important to choose a therapist who has experience working with women with breast cancer. Many fine therapists are skilled in other areas but are quite uninformed about breast cancer and its treatment. You are looking for someone who can help you explore and understand your feelings, but also someone who is educated about the medical world you are entering. You don't need to spend some of your valuable therapy time explaining about radiation or chemotherapy side effects, and you do not want to work with a therapist who may be poorly informed about cancer and may, because of this, frighten you unnecessarily. Feel free to ask your doctor or nurse or other health practitioner for a referral to a therapist whom they know to be helpful in situations like yours. You could also call the social work department of your hospital and ask to speak with their oncology social worker. If your hospital does not have such a specialist, try calling a large teaching hospital nearby. It doesn't matter whether you are receiving your medical care there or not; an oncology social worker can still meet with you or refer you to other therapists in the community. If there is a local breast cancer hotline, they may also be a source of therapy referrals. Finally, you can try calling one of the national organizations for suggestions (see the resources section).

We believe that participating in a breast cancer support group can be the very best way to help yourself. No one can understand what you are going through as well as others on the same journey. Many women are resistant to the idea of joining a group because they fear that hearing others' experiences will make them depressed or frightened. Other women who have never been part of a support or therapy group before may be uncertain of what to expect or may feel uncomfortable with the idea in general. Choosing the right group can be just as important as choosing the right doctors. There are different philosophies about group composition, but we feel strongly that you should look for a group for women newly diagnosed or currently in first-time treatment. In her practice, Hester facilitates several different breast cancer support groups designed to meet the needs of women at different points in the experience. The group for newly diagnosed women is an excellent place to feel understood and less alone, to gather a lot of information about treatment choices or coping with side effects, and to talk about job issues and family concerns. In the right group, while there should be ample opportunity for the expression of all kinds of feelings, on balance, there will be more laughter than tears.

David Spiegel, a psychiatrist at Stanford University, published an important study in 1989 about the positive effect of support groups on the longevity of women with breast cancer. Although his groups were all for women who had metastatic breast cancer, he found that those women who were in support groups lived longer than those who were not. Although these studies have not been duplicated in women with early breast cancer, even in the absence of solid data, it seems reasonable to think the conclusions would be similar. Many studies have documented the positive impact of good social supports for individuals with all kinds of cancer, and there is no social support better than the right group.

There are a number of places to ask about groups. The suggestions we made earlier about how to find a therapist would all apply here, too. Additionally, programs such as the Wellness Community or Gilda's Place offer a number of support groups. Ask whether the groups are professionally led or are peer support groups. Ask who the participants are, and particularly ask about their *stage* of illness. It is our bias that no one's needs are best served by being in a group comprised of women who are dealing with all stages of breast cancer. You would be unnecessarily frightened, as women who are very ill are dealing with different issues than those you currently face.

## Finding Support: Religious Resources

All over the world, when the trauma of serious illness strikes, many people instinctively turn first for guidance and solace to their own religious group, whether the traditional, institutional type, or some newer, hybridized variety. If you are a member of a church, mosque, or synagogue, you will probably seek the counsel of your own clergy, with whom you already have had a prior relationship. Many, if not most, professional clergy have had training in the area of pastoral counseling and will know how to listen to your fears and concerns and/or those of your husband, partner, or close friend. What both of you want is to be reassured that your feelings of confusion, anxiety, anger, and terror constitute a normal, usual response at this time. Your clergy member will want to reassure you and may also feel the need to tell you that everything will be all right. *Please note* that although on one level you want desperately to be told that, indeed, everything will be all right, on another level, you will be suspicious of such a message, since you know that no human being—clergy or physician—can truly guarantee this.

You need a sympathetic ear and advice about how to deal with several issues simultaneously: your own feelings and those of other family members, including perhaps your parents, siblings, children, and friends. You may not feel up to the emotional requirements of dealing with so many people all at once. Both you and your partner may need advice about how best to inform family and friends; your clergy member should be able to help you sort this out and may also connect you to leaders within your community who stand willing to organize other members to help you in the weeks and months ahead.

You and your partner will most likely want to have your intense, almost overwhelming feelings validated by your religious leader. S/he should respond to your concerns by saying either "I know how you feel" (*only if* s/he truly does from personal experience) or "I can imagine how you must be feeling." Most people we know resent the presumption of another person *assuming* s/he knows how you feel—even a professional clergy or physician—unless s/he has actually lived through a similar crisis. Even professional training does not entitle other people to assume that they really know how you are feeling; the truth is that, unless they have had the same experience themselves (either personally or through an immediate family member or close relative), they really do *not* know what you are going through.

For those who are comforted by the strength of their own beliefs, their already established habits of personal prayer will provide crucial support. What had previously furnished a familiar, stabilizing ritual will now, in time of personal crisis, provide a soothing refuge and a pathway toward healing. You will come to realize, and value, the difference between the concept of cure and that of healing. *One can be cured without actually healing, even as one can be helped to heal without actually being cured.*

For others who are not in the habit of daily or frequent prayer, the structure of a familiar religious service within one's own tradition and house of affiliation can be very comforting at this time. Such services may provide a level of grounding and connection to a community of worshipers that offers much-needed comfort. In addition, many religious groups offer specialized services of healing to their congregants on a weekly or monthly basis. Many people find these services to be particularly helpful.

Even the least religious among us might be surprised by the force of the sudden urge to communicate with a higher power or a divine force, in whatever way we may conceive of this. Frequently the usual motivation is to try and strike a bargain. When you are feeling very stressed, and sometimes desperate, you may find yourself pleading and begging with a divine power you have repudiated for many years. You may be truly stunned by the force of your need to feel that you are being heard and listened to and that this, your most urgent request, is being received. This may well be the first time in your life since your childhood that you are asking wholeheartedly for a reprieve—literally, a new lease on life—and the chance to continue living.

notes

# gathering information/
# *choosing your team*

**In the immediate** aftermath of hearing that you have breast cancer, you may find it is difficult to think clearly and make the choices that will influence the rest of your treatment. You may be completely satisfied with the doctor or hospital where you heard the diagnosis, or you may wish to consider other possibilities. There are a few things to remember in your selection of a treatment center. While it is usually easiest to have all your care coordinated in one facility, it is also possible to have different parts of your treatment at different places. You should consider carefully both the need for the best care you can get and the logistics of your life as you move through the months of active treatment.

This period is the very hardest time emotionally. You will feel better after all the medical information has been gathered, after you have met with all of your doctors, and after the treatment decisions have been made. If you are managing to get through your day now, you are doing fine, and you can count on feeling stronger, saner, and less out of control in the future.

Do take someone with you to all of your consultations. You will not remember most of what is said to you, and your companion's ears and memory will be extremely valuable. Prepare ahead! Take written questions with you and have your companion take notes during the consultation. Some doctors are glad to have you tape your meeting; some object to this practice.

In our system of health care, some decisions will likely be made for you based on your medical insurance. Most policies, especially most managed care plans, limit the number of doctors you can see. They may also limit their coverage to doctors who are on their list of approved specialists. If there is a specialist in your area whom you especially want to consult and who is not covered under your plan, it is worth a call to ask if a special referral/exception may be made for a second opinion visit. If the answer is no, it might still be worth it to you to pay out of pocket for a single visit. If you decide to do so, inquire at the physician's office whether there are ways to minimize the bill. For example, you can avoid having any blood work or other laboratory tests done there; if those results are part of the consultation, they can always be sent to the specialist from your usual health care provider at a later date.

After talking with your doctors, you may decide that you want to get a second opinion. Most insurance companies will pay for this. Occasionally it even makes sense to seek a third opinion; this situation would most likely arise if each of two physicians recommends a different course of treatment and you wish to find a "tiebreaker." In any case, you should prepare yourself both mentally and emotionally to become actively involved in the process of choosing your treatment.

Cancer care is delivered in several different kinds of settings, and you may feel more comfortable in one than in the others. With the exception of certain clinical trials, which are available only at participating cancer programs, you can receive the same treatment at each place, and your decision may be based on other factors.

## Treatment Sites

Consider the following possible treatment settings:

- Academic or teaching hospitals are likely to have the biggest names in your community on their staffs and to have access to current clinical trials.
- Community cancer centers may be located closer to your home and may also participate in some research programs.
- Private oncology practices may be the most convenient, and you may prefer the small size of the whole operation. This would feel comparable to going to your regular doctor's office.
- Combinations of the above exist in many areas. For example, you may be able to meet with your oncologist in her/his private office away from the hospital and receive your chemotherapy either there or in a hospital-based unit.

Breast cancer care varies in complexity depending upon the clinical circumstances. Most situations require an integrated approach involving a number of specialists:

- A breast surgeon, who does the initial biopsy (unless that has already been done by another surgeon) and then the second surgery of either wide excision/partial mastectomy (also referred to as a lumpectomy) or mastectomy. Both of these definitive surgeries are likely to include an axillary node sampling.
- A plastic surgeon, if you are having a mastectomy and considering reconstruction.
- A radiation oncologist, if you are having a lumpectomy followed by radiation. Some women also have radiation following a mastectomy.
- A medical oncologist, who plans and delivers your chemotherapy or hormone therapy.

As one oncologist says to his new patients, "This is a long-term relationship." You will be followed by all of these people for a long time, and you must feel comfortable with and trust them. Your medical oncologist will be the long-term captain of your care team, so it is especially important that you have a good relationship with him or her.

Many large hospitals have something like an interdisciplinary breast clinic. Scheduling an appointment in one of these centers, even if you don't anticipate receiving all of your care at that hospital, can be an excellent and efficient way of gathering information. In a single visit, you will be able to meet with a surgeon, a radiation oncologist, and a medical oncologist.

Often a radiologist (who would be expert at reading mammograms and other radiographic tests) and a pathologist are also part of the team, although you probably will not meet them. The advantage to one of these clinics is that in a single day you will be able to hear from each of the treating physicians and leave with a clear recommendation and/or treatment plans. You can then decide whether to take this information back to another doctor or whether to continue your care at that facility. The disadvantage of this system is that the single day can be a long, exhausting, and stressful one.

Remember that you may find it hard to like someone who is giving you so much bad news. Many women initially dislike their doctors, yet end up liking them enormously. Unless you have a really bad experience with someone, you probably should give him/her a second chance.

All of this sounds harder than it really is. You have already heard the worst news, the fact that you have breast cancer, and you heard those words from a physician. If you do only what your first doctor suggests, the chances are good that you will be referred to specialists who are respected in your community. However, since breast cancer is a potentially life-threatening illness, and since you want to do everything possible to ensure the very best care for yourself, it is wise to select your medical team thoughtfully and carefully. If you don't know where to go, ask others. The breast cancer network is far-reaching, and you will quickly find that you have resources you were previously unaware of. You probably already know some women who have had breast cancer; talk with them and they will refer you to others. Ask these women about their doctors and about their level of satisfaction with their care. Would they make the same decisions if they were starting out now? You can call one of the breast cancer organizations listed in the resources section of this book. They will probably not be able to suggest individual physicians, but they can give you a list of cancer centers and accredited oncologists in your community.

Here are some things to remember as you choose your medical team:

- First and foremost, you are looking for the best doctors in your area with whom you feel comfortable.
- Most likely your medical insurance plan will place some limits on your choices. Your doctors will need to be on their list of approved providers/specialists.
- Geography matters. Although it is certainly worth traveling a reasonable distance for better care, remember that you will be spending a fair amount of time with doctors and treatments in the site you select. Since one overall goal is to make your life easier, not harder, whenever possible, you might want to consider geographic location very carefully.
- Trust your gut. Remembering that it is hard to like the messenger of bad tidings, pay attention to your reaction to the doctors with whom you are speaking. Do they treat you respectfully? Do they spend enough time to answer your questions? Do they talk to you and not to your spouse or partner? Do they tell you how to reach them or their coverage at any time, and do they suggest the best way to ask them questions at times other than during office visits?

- Ask to tour the treatment area. It will *not* be as scary as you imagine, and different practices are set up in different ways. Would you be more comfortable in a large and airy space, where you can see other patients and the nurses at all times, or would you prefer a small and private room away from others?

- Ask who administers the chemotherapy and whether you can be introduced. Most often chemotherapy is given by skilled and experienced oncology nurses; some oncologists, however, do it themselves. One way is not better than the other; they are just different systems.

- Ask about available support services. Is there an oncology social worker on site? Can you and your family meet with her or him? Are there support groups? Peer support programs? Educational materials? Resources for your family—your partner, husband, children?

- Several of us have found it helpful while living through this crisis to encourage different family members to attend age-appropriate support or focus groups. Even when children don't want to go to such meetings initially, they almost always feel surprisingly positive afterwards. With children, it is important to find groups divided by age; the issues most important to elementary school children are quite different from those most pressing to high school students. Even though your kids may be reluctant or resistant to going the first time, most of them will find solace in being with peers (even though they will be strangers) who are dealing with a parent's cancer. They find it a relief to be able to talk about a range of deep-seated fears and feelings that they are reluctant to discuss with friends whose parents are healthy. If you choose to involve your children in a support program or group, you must inquire about the family situations of other children in the group! Just as it would be frightening for you to attend a group with women who are dying from breast cancer, it would be completely overwhelming and destructive to your children's well-being to be in a group with others who have a terminally ill parent. Be sure of this before you send your children anywhere!

■ Having made a careful decision, trust yourself and trust your new doctors.

## Complementary Therapies

Many women facing cancer treatment are interested in complementary or alternative therapies. Traditional or Western treatments for breast cancer include surgery, radiation, chemotherapy, hormone therapy, and biologic therapy. All other treatments can be considered complementary. Since we feel strongly that there is far-reaching and impressive data to support the value of traditional medical treatments for breast cancer and no comparable set of data exists for complementary therapies, we implore you to use these other modalities *in addition to*, rather than in lieu of, standard medical care. This is the reason that we are referring to them as complementary rather than alternative treatments. Having said that, we recognize that many women are motivated to do everything possible to help themselves, and that some believe that non-Western health traditions have much to offer.

Frequently, this is also an area where friends may give advice. You may find yourself the recipient of many articles and books espousing one or another treatment, diet, or program to cure cancer. Of course you may find all this interesting and welcome. If you do not, one strategy can be to ask someone to screen your mail, setting aside all such literature. You can then look at it later if you wish.

There is often controversy about the value of these treatments. This is because alternative, or complementary, therapies often have not been subjected to carefully designed clinical trials. A clinical trial is a research study designed to evaluate the effectiveness or value of a particular treatment. In the context of treatment for early breast cancer, any option offered under a clinical trial would be considered to be at least as effective as the prevailing standard treatment for the same condition. On the other hand, most standard treatments for breast cancer have been subjected to such clinical trials and have therefore accrued substantial scientific data to support their value.

One useful distinction is between the hope that a complementary therapy will cure your cancer and the hope that a complementary therapy will improve your quality of life during or after treatment. There is a big difference between a treatment's shrinking a tumor and a treatment's effect on nausea, fatigue, or general well-being. Many women undergoing chemotherapy and/or radiation find some symptom relief and psychological benefit from one or more of these therapies.

Examples of complementary therapies are acupuncture, massage, meditation and visualization, hypnosis, herbal medicine, vitamin therapy, naturopathy, and chiropractic. You can talk with practitioners about the goals of their particular therapies. In general, some women believe that their overall sense of well-being—in particular their nausea and fatigue—has been helped by some of these treatments. Some also believe that their immune system has been boosted, and therefore their body's mechanisms for fighting cancer have been helped.

It is vital that you inform all of your caregivers, conventional doctors as well as complementary therapists, of everything you are doing. Even if they disagree with some of your choices, you are protecting yourself with full disclosure. You must tell your doctors about anything you are ingesting (for example, herbs, teas, vitamins), as there is some evidence that certain substances may interfere with your chemotherapy or radiation treatments. Many doctors prefer that you wait until your treatments are completed before taking these supplements.

It is unlikely that you can safely assume that your doctors and other health care providers will be well informed about these other options. Western medical training and experience does not emphasize them, and there have not been controlled studies to evaluate their efficacy. Having said this, we note the trend in medical education to include courses of teaching about complementary and alternative therapies. Physicians are increasingly being asked about these options by their patients and need to be able to advise them in an informed and thoughtful manner. In a recent study conducted by physicians at Harvard Medical School and published in the *Journal of the American Medical Association*, (*week of September 1, 1998*), the authors state that "as a profession, physicians will increasingly be expected to advise patients who use, seek or demand complementary and alternative therapies." The study was based on the 117 medical schools replying to their original survey, which had been mailed to all 125 schools listed in *The Directory of American Medical Education*. The study concludes that in the future, more medical schools will offer courses in complementary and alternative therapies (presently 64 percent of the 117 replying already do) in response to increased patient demand for "a physician who is solidly grounded in conventional, orthodox medicine and is also knowledgeable about the values and limitations of alternative treatments."

Often oncology social workers or oncology nurses will be better informed about these treatments and may be able to refer you to practitioners in your community. There are other ways to find nontraditional practitioners, and we list some of those organizations in our resources section. Talking with other women who have had breast cancer is also a good way to learn about trusted practitioners in your area.

It is smart to talk with a practitioner before starting his or her treatments, just as you would when selecting any doctor or health care provider. Feel free to ask as many questions as you would of your conventional doctors. Ask especially about their previous experience in treating women with breast cancer and what they believe the impact of their care will be on your chemotherapy or radiation treatments. Be advised that most medical insurance companies do not cover complementary therapies, although there are a few exceptions. For example, chiropractors are more often included in coverage, and a few policies cover acupuncture. It is worth a phone call to your insurance carrier ahead of time to determine what might be covered.

Many women find that during the first weeks or months of breast cancer, they are very interested in any treatment that might help them. Newly diagnosed women may embark upon an ambitious program of careful diet and other modalities of care. These same women oftentimes lose interest in these activities, decide that they do not wish to spend so much time, energy, and money focusing on cancer, and resume their usual life patterns and habits. Once again, you will find your own way and make choices that fit you and your life. Do not feel that, on the one hand, you must partake of multiple complementary therapies or that, on the other, you must avoid them all.

At the very least, it is worth knowing that these other therapies exist. If you like, you might consider how to use them as adjuncts to your medical care, once you have discussed these possible choices thoroughly with your physicians. Reserve the right to change your mind as time passes.

notes

# notes

practical tips on
*getting yourself ready*

# Between Diagnosis and Treatment

- Remember this is as bad as it gets emotionally. You *will* feel better.
- Be kind to yourself. You are under an enormous amount of stress.
- Find a breast cancer support group and get there. This may be the one exception to the general rule to try to minimize your commitments. Nothing will help you as much as being with other women who are living, and living well, with breast cancer.
- If you don't already know how to say no, now is the time to start practicing.
- If you don't already know how to say yes, now is also the time to start practicing.
- Accept offers of assistance if you think they will really be helpful. When you are not sure, tell others you will get back to them and keep a list of people who have offered

to help; there will probably be things for them to do at a later date.

- Just because you will find it interesting later, make a list for yourself of people who you anticipate will help and people who you don't think would ever consider doing anything for you. Put it away for a year. You will be surprised.

- Start keeping a list by your kitchen phone of things friends can do for you (for example, cook a dinner, pick up your dry cleaning, drive a child to soccer practice, walk the dog).

- If you have young children, make arrangements for someone to help care for them while you are in the hospital and also when you come home.

- Look for laughter: movies, silly TV shows, books (including comic books or cartoons)—anything that makes you laugh out loud.

- "Retail therapy" also helps many people. We can't recommend one woman's purchase of a new Saab convertible to everyone, but a new quilt for the bed or fresh flowers or that dress you have been wanting may be in order now.

- Do whatever gives you pleasure, whether it's cooking special dishes, gardening, playing sports, curling up and reading, or taking mini excursions with your partner, your child(ren), or a close friend. Spend time doing what you enjoy!

■ ■ ■

# Clothing

- Soft, front-closing bras are much more comfortable after surgery than regular back-fastening bras; when trying these on, make sure they are loose.

- Try athletic bras.

- Consider buying a couple of soft, loose camisoles or undershirts. You may prefer these against your skin before you are ready to put on a bra. If you are having a mastectomy without reconstruction, it is possible to buy camisoles with pockets for a prosthesis to wear during this time.

- Buy some soft, comfortable nighties in your favorite pretty colors; loose, front-buttoning ones are the kind to choose. It will be difficult to raise your arms or to struggle in and out of tight garments. Look at pajamas, too— even if you haven't worn them since childhood. They are easier in the hospital.

- Think about buying or requesting a bed jacket (yes, like your grandmother's) because it will keep you warm without getting tangled up under the bedclothes the way a long bathrobe will.

- If you are having a mastectomy without reconstruction, take a large, loose, button-down-the-front shirt or a sweatshirt to wear home. You may not want to use even a temporary prosthesis that soon.

- If you are having a mastectomy without reconstruction, you will find, unless you are extremely large breasted, that dressing in layers can minimize or even eliminate the need for a prosthesis. Try vests, shawls, and long scarves that hang around your neck and down your chest.

- A number of national catalogs sell appropriate clothing. Look in some of your favorites.
- Buy, borrow, or request a couple of small (baby-sized) pillows. These will come in handy after surgery for supporting your sore arm and side. Some women also use them between their chest and the seat belt of their car for a while after surgery.

## Meals

- Freeze some meals and appealing snacks and treats ahead of your surgery. Accept food that friends prepare for you; use some and freeze the rest.
- Ask your friends for help with meals the first few days you are home from the hospital. They will be glad to help out. It is easier for people to comply when they are asked to perform a specific task.
- Explore the availability of home-delivered meals. There are restaurants, catering services, and small businesses that provide this helpful service.
- This is not a time to diet. Eat what you crave.

## Planning for Your Hospital Stay

The reality of medicine today is that you may not spend even a single night in the hospital throughout your breast cancer experience. We have even heard of women being discharged on the same day that they have undergone mastectomies. If you know that you are not feeling well enough to go home, say so and say so loudly. You may need to make more of a scene than seems comfortable, but just say no!

- If you are sensitive to noises, pack your Walkman and favorite tapes. Consider using earplugs; you can buy them in any drugstore.
- Even if you are not sensitive to noises, music can be nice to have. Bring something you enjoy listening to.
- You may be sharing a hospital room—an eye mask helps you nap if you're sensitive to lights.
- While hospital gowns aren't beautiful, they are practical because they have shoulder snaps or ties. They may be easier to use for the first few days.
- Leave favorite pieces of jewelry, watches, and rings at home. Your family can bring them when they visit.
- Bring your cosmetics, favorite cologne, postcards, or notecards you like to look at and some family pictures. Soft, stretchy headbands or pretty barrettes can help keep your hair under control until you can wash it. You might want to bring some dry (powder-type) "shampoo" to fill in until you can take a shower. Bring (or ask someone to bring in) a blow dryer.
- If you are going to be in the hospital for several days, consider taking some nail polish and asking a friend (after your surgery) to give you a manicure and/or pedicure.

■   ■   ■

- Tuck some magazines into your hospital kit. It is even possible that you will have the energy to read a book, but bring only light and entertaining reading.
- Bring your own pillow in a pretty case.
- It is okay to bring your favorite quilt, too.
- If you live alone, you may need help at home for a few days. There are resources in every community. Ask your nurse or social worker. Some hospitals have programs prior to your admission that enable you to get this information. When you are given the information about your surgery, ask whether there is someone with whom you can speak about home care assistance.

notes

notes

# personal *relationships*

# Partners

**A diagnosis of** breast cancer is almost as hard on a partner as on the woman directly affected. Generally speaking, men find it more difficult than women to express their feelings, to ask for and accept help. It is also common that the attention of family and friends is focused on the patient; few people think to ask the patient's husband how he is doing. Breast cancer is a family disease, and a husband may be more directly involved than anyone else.

He may be expected to listen to your fears and grief, to take on some of your usual responsibilities, to accompany you to doctors' appointments, to support and reassure your children. Like you, he is sad and scared and unsure how to best help you and your family. Unlike you, and this may be difficult to contemplate, he must also worry about how to care for your family if you should not survive this illness. The burdens of these real worries are enormous, and many men are ill prepared to cope with them. Husbands of women with breast cancer often talk about how overwhelmed they are feeling, and how much they miss their wives "as they used to be." No one expects you to pretend that you are carefree, but it will help your husband if you can sometimes focus on the happiness of the moment.

The best advice, again, is open and honest communication. Tell him how you are feeling. Let him know what frightens you. Ask him to hold you. Talk about the changes you may be experiencing in your body and your libido. Remember the joys you have shared and plan for the future together.

Encourage your husband to find someone he can talk to. He will feel that he can't share with you all of what he is feeling; he worries about burdening you and protecting you. Some hospitals have support groups for husbands; ask what is available to help him. Suggest that he continue with activities that have been fun for him in the past; playing golf or fishing or going out with friends will help him manage the harder days.

Most husbands rise to the occasion and provide unlimited love and support to their wives. Some, however, do not. If your husband seems angry or rejecting or preoccupied or otherwise unavailable to you, remember that what you are seeing is likely *his* problem and *his* issues. Try to talk with him. If you cannot, find your support elsewhere and encourage him to do likewise.

We recognize that there are other kinds of partnerships in the world. Many who are not husbands may experience the same feelings as their married brothers. Newer boyfriends often become more loving and involved and appreciative of what you share together. Lesbian couples experience all of the same feelings and may have some concerns about how others will react to them. The incidence of breast cancer is even higher in the lesbian community, so most lesbian women will already be familiar with the problem. This may be a moment when the fact that your partner is also a woman means that it is easier for her to truly empathize and understand what you are going through. There are support groups in many areas specifically for lesbian women and their partners facing breast cancer.

## Concerns of Husbands

Some husbands have told us they were surprised that from the very beginning they felt they were unimportant to the doctors and other caregivers trying to help their wives. Some of them had a difficult time getting used to the fact that for the duration of their wives' treatment, the doctors attending their wives, as well as the entire hospital staff, were focused completely on their wives' well-being and did not ever acknowledge the husbands' needs. This is, of course, uncomfortable and unfortunate. Full attention and support is often focused on the patient, and to some extent, this is completely appropriate. Husbands/partners may need to look elsewhere to find support for themselves. It is not really reasonable at this time to lean on your wife. She needs to lean on you. Husbands/partners need to talk with their own family (perhaps siblings or parents) and friends.

Husbands/partners often experience a total sense of loss of control from the first minute of the diagnosis. Events unfurl extremely fast. Appointments are often made for tests and for surgeries without any attempt to consult with them in any meaningful way. This, too, is less than ideal, but the realities of busy hospitals are that appointments are made without much consideration of anyone's schedule. The emphasis is on getting the patient what he/she needs as quickly as possible. In most cases, the husbands had confidence in the doctors helping their wives, and they trusted the doctors' judgment and were content to stay in the shadows. However, some husbands want to emphasize the point that if you or your partner feel that something is wrong with the way the diagnosis is being made or the treatment is being planned, you must reassert some measure of control and press the doctors for further explanations. In the rare case that you feel something is very wrong, you must discuss your feelings with your husband and get a second opinion. You both must feel comfortable with the physicians you ultimately choose. Remember, however, that you are the patient. If you don't have confidence in the doctor, find another one that you trust. Don't allow yourselves to be stampeded by the medical establishment.

In all likelihood, some member of your family will have an especially hard time coming to grips with your illness. It may be one of your children or it may be your mother or father. A partner can provide immeasurable help by spending time with this child or with whoever most needs extra attention.

Some husbands have told us that their children assume that the death of their mother is a real possibility. Let them talk about their fears and their feelings with both of you if that feels right to you both. It may be that your wife cannot emotionally handle too much of this conversation at this time, and you can help by being the primary support person for your kids. Do not put them down. Do not give them pat statements that everything will turn out all right. They will sense that you are not being honest with them. If your doctors have painted an optimistic picture to you, share this with your children. Explain that in nearly all cases the cancer can be arrested, and that chemotherapy and radiation therapy are meant to kill all of the remaining cancer cells. Let them know that you too are scared. You will be surprised at how they will immediately want to help you. Let them try to help you; you will both feel better. Remember that all families are different and yours will react in ways appropriate for them.

Your husband's male friends may have a difficult time providing him with any real emotional support. They may stare at their shoes when they ask how you are doing, clearly indicating that they are not really able to say anything further. If your husband is lucky, he will have one or two friends who will seek him out—perhaps over the telephone—and ask how he is feeling. Your husband can try telling them how he feels and see if they pick up on it. If he is lucky enough to have male friends capable of real empathy, he is very fortunate.

## Concerns of Single Women

Women who do not have life partners may experience special stresses and worries as they move through the experience of having breast cancer. Remember that being married or having a committed, significant other is no guarantee of receiving unconditional and constant support. Many single women have friends who serve as family during this crisis in better ways than "real" family members would do. You may have to think creatively about who can be asked to help with what, but be assured that friends are waiting to be told what they can do for you.

Single women may also worry about how they will continue in, or how they can rejoin, the social world with the physical changes and emotional issues which breast cancer brings. It has been our experience that women who have had breast cancer, whether they have two breasts or not, will have the same success with men that they have always had. We have even been told by a few women that "men find me interesting . . . I'm a little different from most of the women out there." Any man who is worth having will appreciate and love you whatever your breasts look like. As someone said, "We all have scars in life; ours are just more visible than some others."

This is not intended to minimize what you might be going through right now. It is hard enough to deal with the dating world when you are feeling at the top of your game. When you are feeling vulnerable and scared and less than attractive, it may feel overwhelming. We wish that we could reassure you that your social scene will not be different after breast cancer than it was before; but of course, we cannot guarantee this. However, you might be pleasantly surprised to find it may actually improve.

This story may help. Jennifer was a never-married woman in her mid-forties at the time of her diagnosis. She had a mastectomy and chemotherapy; two years later, she had a recurrence in a regional lymph node. She had just joined a dating service and found herself on the phone with a match the evening before she was to begin radiation treatment to her neck. It turned out that the man with whom she had been matched was a physician who worked in the emergency room of the hospital where she was to receive radiation. He suggested that they meet at the hospital after her first treatment. Now, several years later, she is well, and they are married.

## Multicultural Issues

Women from nonwhite middle-class cultures bring their own experiences and expectations to breast cancer. For example, in the Haitian community, it is still sometimes considered inappropriate to even talk about breasts and quite shameful to have cancer, especially in the breast. The main reason for the higher mortality rate from cancer in minority communities is later diagnosis. This is due to less good access to medical care, poor or no medical insurance, less information about self-care and health, and less comfort in general with talking about cancer or sexualized body parts.

If you are from a minority community, you have the same rights as anyone else to the best care and best support services. You may not feel comfortable being an assertive health care consumer if you have been raised to believe that any authority figure, and especially a doctor, is always right. You may find it harder to ask questions or go after a second opinion. Remember that your first responsibility is to yourself and that you deserve the very best care you can find.

There are intrinsic supports in the community that can be helpful to you now. Many African-American churches have support groups for cancer patients or women's alliances that can help with transportation, child care, meals, or whatever you need. Call the local office of your American Cancer Society and ask what is available in your own community.

If you do not feel comfortable and respected in your hospital or doctor's office, speak up. Bring a friend or family member with you and ask for what you need. You might also want to contact the National Black Women's Health Project in Washington, D.C. (see the resources section).

## Children

For most of us, the most painful and frightening aspect of the whole breast cancer experience is associated with our children and our mothering. Whatever else we think about parenting, we assume that we will be around to give our children safe passage to adulthood. It is absolutely devastating to be confronted with the possibility that we might not be able to carry through that basic promise. Mothers of both younger and older children experience these feelings, and the sadness can be so great that we can't find the words to express it. Women who have not yet completed their families find that they too are struggling with an enormous loss and grief as they confront the possible end of a life's dream. For the sake of our children and our families, we must find ways to understand our powerful feelings, to communicate with one another, and to believe in the real probabilities of our long and healthy lives.

There are a few basic themes for how best to help our children cope during the time of our diagnosis and treatment for breast cancer.

- Never lie to your children. If you don't know the answer to a question, say so.
- If your child/ren ask you if you are going to die from your breast cancer, it is honest and right to say no. Most women with breast cancer do well. If it eventually turns out that you are not so fortunate, there will be plenty of time to talk about that and to prepare your children. No one ever dropped dead from breast cancer, and right now what your children need most is to be reassured and comforted. Fears about your future health belong in discussions between you, your husband, and your adult family and friends, not in conversations with your young children. They have more than enough to deal with just now.
- Explain what is happening in words age-appropriate for each child. Children are excellent observers but terrible interpreters of what they see around them. Even though you may be trying to protect them by not talking about your experience, their fantasies are probably much worse than the reality. A good model of communication can be the way you have talked with them about sex. In both cases, you are using honest and age-appropriate language and hoping to make the subject safe and acceptable for future conversations.
- Try to keep their lives and their routines as normal as possible. For more than ten years now, Hester has been

part of a longitudinal study of children of women with breast cancer. Regardless of the age of the children or the specifics of the mother's illness, the consistent finding has been that children who are given honest information in age-appropriate language and whose own routines are not disrupted unnecessarily do fine.

- Remember to tell the appropriate person (teacher, guidance counselor, principal, etc.) at the child's school what is happening at home. This also applies to coaches, music teachers, or other adults who are part of the child's life.
- Whatever their ages, your children will take their cues from you. If you are straightforward and positive about your diagnosis and treatment, they will be, too.
- Do not be surprised or hurt if your children quickly become blasé about your diagnosis. This means you are doing a good job!

## Preschool Children

Very young children will not understand the facts and details about what is happening; they will, however, know that something is very wrong. In reaction they may be more clingy and irritable, or conversely, they may be too well behaved and anxious to please. What they need most is reassurance that someone (ideally someone whom they already know and trust) will always be there to care for them and reassurance that they are not responsible or to blame for what has happened. *The normal magical thinking of young children may lead them to believe that their anger or words have caused your illness; tell them directly that this is not so.*

You must also distinguish between your cancer treatment and the more ordinary illnesses that may happen to them. We have heard stories of young children panicked about taking an antibiotic because "mommy's medicine" made her hair fall out! Many mothers worry that their young children will be especially upset if they lose their hair because it is harder to explain the process to them. Our experience has been that preschool children accept their mother's baldness as one more interesting and new thing about the world. One woman said that her three-year-old daughter wanted her to come to nursery school as her show-and-tell exhibit!

## Elementary School Children

Latency age children may have lots of questions. Some children will be more curious than others; try to answer all questions as briefly and honestly as possible. Answer only what you are asked. Remember to think of this the way you would health or sex education. If you do not know the answer, say so.

Children this age also need reassurance that they will be cared for while you are in the hospital or having treatments. They need to know that their daily lives and routines will be disrupted as little as possible. If you will be spending time in the hospital, they may like to have a calendar to mark off the days you will be away. Some might like a special blank book to write or draw in. Others might want to write you notes while you are in the hospital; give them paper, cards, envelopes, and stamps. Frequent short phone calls are a boon.

Invite your children to accompany you to the hospital when you are going for a short appointment. Particularly if you ask your doctor or nurse to suggest a good time for a visit, your children will be welcomed; they will be interested in meeting your caregivers and seeing where you are spending so much time. Children are rarely frightened by the treatment areas; indeed, they are generally quite reassured by seeing them. Their fantasies are much more frightening than the realities.

Mothers may find it disturbing to discover that their children have told all their friends and classmates about the illness or its side effects. Children do not have the same sense of what is private that you do, and your calm management of the situation may enable them to share the news with everyone in a matter-of-fact way. The positive effect of this is likely to be that many people, even some whom you do not know well, will offer to help. Many elementary school classrooms organize dinners for a student's mother undergoing chemotherapy. If you are lucky enough to have this come your way, say yes. Make sure your own child's teacher and classmates know how much you appreciate their help and the efforts of their parents. Write (or draw, depending on the age of the children) a communal note that your child can help you create and might want to read out loud (if s/he feels comfortable doing this), or ask the teacher to do it on your behalf. Alternatively, you might ask your child's teacher to pin your note of thanks up in the classroom or to transcribe it onto the blackboard.

■ ■ ■

## Middle School Children

Preadolescent children can be tough! Like their younger siblings, they may have many questions—or they may not. You may want to talk with them more than they want to talk with you. As long as you repeat the message that you will be available to talk when your son or daughter is ready, you will be leaving the lines of communication open. It is okay to let your older child know that you are sad and frightened; you don't have to hide or deny your feelings in front of your children in an attempt to protect them. They will be confused and will think it strange if you do not admit to strong, negative feelings.

Children this age have a strong need to be just like their peers. Having a mother with cancer is different, and they may react with embarrassment and shame. They may have an especially difficult time with the changes in your physical appearance and may ask you to always wear a wig (rather than a hat or scarf) when their friends are around. Preadolescent girls, obviously, may be especially upset by your breast surgery, and preadolescent boys may be totally wordless and embarrassed because of their sexual association with breasts. On the other hand, boys this age may surprise you with their tender naïveté. One of our sons was totally confused when told his mother would need further surgery, in addition to the lumpectomy she had previously had, because he could not even conceive of the possibility of having an entire breast removed. To him this was a permanent, irremovable body part. When the full reality was explained to him and the realization of what this meant registered fully, he suddenly burst into tears.

Middle school children may be furious that you have told their principal or guidance counselor about your diagnosis. You should still tell someone at the school, but it would be smart to ask that he or she not say anything directly to your child. As long as the school knows about the home situation, they will keep a watchful eye out for signs of trouble; they will not need to single out your child, which would certainly cause him or her great embarrassment.

## High School Children

Adolescent children may or may not want to discuss your cancer. They may or may not want to accompany you to the hospital. Some kids this age find the whole disease monumentally embarrassing, and since they are adolescents, what matters most to them is what their friends think. Try to maintain a whimsical tolerance of your teenage son or daughter if at all possible. Underneath the bravado and the posturing, s/he is very frightened and worried about you. Try to find ways to encourage discussion; words may come more easily during a drive to swim practice than in the living room. Do not be afraid to ask your adolescent children for help and to rely on them. They can be very helpful, and although they may sometimes resent being asked to do things for you, in general they will be glad to take care of some family tasks. The obvious warning is don't ask or expect too much—they are, after all, children, not adults.

Adolescent daughters are likely to be worried about their own risk of breast cancer. Whether or not they themselves bring this up, you should do so. It is honest to be optimistic about their future health, and you should say so.

Reassure your children that they can continue to have friends come over once you feel up to the company. Tell them you will not embarrass them on purpose, but make sure that they tell their friends what to expect—for example, Mom may be wearing a hat/turban/wig while she is waiting for her hair to grow in. Mothers of adolescent boys in particular have told us many stories of endearing behavior centered around their parent's baldness. If you are comfortable at home without anything on your head, it is likely that your children will be, too. You may find that your son's friends make a point of rubbing your bald head as they say hello. We have even known a few sons who shaved their own heads in solidarity with their mother, and we heard of one son's entire basketball team doing the same thing as a way of showing support.

## Adult Children

The impact of your cancer on your grown children will be significant. Frequently young adult children—that is to say, those college age or slightly older—may seem quite unconcerned about your diagnosis. This is usually perplexing and even hurtful to the mother, but it may help to know that it is normal. Their apparent nonchalance masks very real worry. They are trying to learn how to be independent of you; this sometimes makes it too difficult to let you know how frightened they are. If this is the case with your children, know that sooner or later, they will express the true depth of their concern for you.

Daughters worry both about you and about themselves; their risk of breast cancer does increase a little with your diagnosis, and they will need to be extra careful about monthly breast self-exams and, after the age of thirty-five, about mammograms. As mothers, we may find it painful to face the fact that we have inadvertently, through no fault of our own, slightly increased our daughters' breast cancer risks. Remind yourselves that your daughters will be likely to take special care of themselves, since their awareness has been heightened. Also, remember that real advances are being made in prevention and treatment, and we can hope that the incidence of breast cancer will be much reduced in our daughters.

In thinking about the impact of breast cancer on your children, remember that this is not just a disease that affects female body parts. Breast cancer, like many other cancers, affects the whole person and her family. In some real sense, the whole family can feel stricken by this insidious disease.

Although both sons and daughters will be strongly impacted by their mothers' struggle with breast cancer, adolescent and young adult daughters may be most painfully affected. Unlike their brothers, they must carry the added burden of wondering if they, too, will become victims of this disease in the future. Most of them know that their statistical likelihood is greater than that of their girlfriends whose mothers are disease-free. Remember that their statistical risk is increased only a little. Your diagnosis absolutely does not sentence them to a future cancer. Each young woman has to work through these fears—acknowledging, confronting, and discussing these issues in her own way and on her own terms.

These issues become particularly acute at times of major

**woman to woman**

life changes and transitions, such as finishing high school, beginning a new job, and/or going off to college. Although these transition periods are also very stressful for young men as well, for a variety of reasons (some societal, some cultural, some individual), young women who are daughters of women newly diagnosed with breast cancer may have an especially difficult time with these life passages.

During the years between eighteen and twenty-two our daughters typically strike out on their own, move away from home, and become independent adults, developing their own identities and their own lifestyles. However, our daughters may feel more than the usual level of conflict during this normal process because they are coping simultaneously with unusual demands on their time, attention, and energy from their moms who are ill back home, usually in a different physical location and often at a considerable distance. They feel conflicted, torn between wanting to be available (both physically and emotionally) and wanting to separate and live their own, individual lives.

We have heard college age and adult sons and daughters of mothers with breast cancer describe the fear of being excluded from the real situation at home and their anger when they discover that certain details have indeed been kept from them during their absence in order to spare them unnecessary worry. We have also known many who opt to maintain some distance and separation from what is happening at home. As is the case with their younger siblings, most college age and young adult children will do fine as long as they are given honest information and the chance to participate or not, as they choose.

Some adult children may try a combination of different coping mechanisms, sometimes fully engaging in social situations, sometimes retreating and withdrawing from peers, except those who also have a parent struggling with a life-threatening disease. At other times, these young adults might find solace in rituals that provide comfort; some are based in conventional religious practices and others are less traditional in origin. Still other adult children might display different forms of rebellion, such as a predilection for unusual risk-taking activities.

Having a mother (or father) who goes through cancer is likely to impact significantly how a young person thinks about, and shapes, major life decisions. The extent to which this medical crisis affects the maturing children depends on whether or not the cancer treatment succeeds in vaulting the patient into remission. In most cases when the treatment is, or appears to be, successful, the children go on about their business. Obviously, when a family is not so fortunate, and the patient's condition worsens, the effect is profoundly different.

In any case, the experience of living with a parent who has cancer produces an unusually early awareness of mortality in the children. Such an increased level of sensitivity and anxiety often influences acutely the choices young adult children make about their work, careers, and relationships—choices that may set them apart from their peers.

Adult children who live far away from home may feel guilty about the distance and their inability to be of much practical help to you. Encourage frequent telephone calls and plan visits as you can. A good time for a trip home might be after your surgery, when you could use some extra assistance for a few days. You might also plan time together when your treatment will be over. This will be something for both of you to look forward to.

They may want to accompany you to an appointment with your doctor(s) and may have questions to ask. It is extremely important to respect their maturity by including them, when it seems appropriate, and by fully sharing information about your diagnosis and treatment.

Mothers of adult children do not have to worry about who would raise their children should they die, but they otherwise have all the same feelings as mothers of young children do. None of us wants to face the possibility of leaving our children prematurely. We all hope to live long enough to see our young adult children settled, and we look forward to celebrating important milestones with them.

## *inviolable rules*

- NEVER LIE TO YOUR CHILDREN.
- ALWAYS LOVE THEM unconditionally and reassure them that your illness is not anyone's fault. Let them know repeatedly that you will *always* love them, even when you do not like or appreciate their behavior at all times.

notes

# making *decisions*

**You may need** to decide simultaneously about both local (mastectomy or lumpectomy/radiation) and systemic (chemotherapy or hormone therapy) treatments. You will feel confused and overwhelmed. Again, remember that your best resources are your doctors, other women who have gone through this, and information from books, medical journals, and magazines. Again, it may be important to limit what you read. Much of what is available in bookstores and libraries and on the web can be overwhelming and frightening. Read only what is relevant to you and your particular situation. Try hard not to read ahead about possible future difficulties! It is not helpful to create extra anxiety about every possible thing that might happen to you.

## Surgical Choices (Local Treatment)

You have already had a biopsy. The primary treatment for breast cancer is almost always surgery, and you may have choices:

- Breast conservation or lumpectomy, in which only the tumor and surrounding tissue are removed
- Mastectomy with or without reconstruction

## Axillary Node Dissections

Either of the surgery options is likely to include an axillary node dissection, in which some of the nodes under your arm are removed by your surgeon to be studied by the pathologist(s). The pathologist's examination of these tissues gives information about the stage and prognosis of the breast cancer. This information is considered in making additional treatment decisions, such as chemotherapy and hormonal therapy and possible radiation treatments to the axilla (armpit) and breast or chest wall. Side effects of an axillary dissection vary among individual women, but may include discomfort, numbness, and/or swelling.

In order to minimize the surgery to be done in the axilla and to diminish possible, unpleasant physical changes, a less invasive surgery has been developed. This procedure is called selective lymph node dissection (SLND) and resection of the sentinel node. This smaller surgery has been offered in some hospitals for several years and has been found to provide all the same important information as the more invasive standard axillary node dissection does.

The sentinel node is the first draining node of a regional lymph node basin. For women with breast cancer, this is most commonly the axilla or underarm area. The theory is that the sentinel node is the first node where cancer cells would lodge if they have traveled through the lymphatics. By removing and testing a sentinel node for cancer cells, your medical team can determine if further surgery is necessary. This is done at the time of definitive surgery for breast cancer. There are two ways the sentinel node can be located. Some surgeons perform one technique or the other, and some use a combination of the two. The first technique uses a radioactive material called technetium (the same tracer used for bone scans), which is injected at the site of the breast tumor. The tracer is then taken up into the lymphatic channels and accumulates in the sentinel node. The surgeon then uses a handheld probe that detects signals from the tracer to locate and identify the node.

Another way to locate the sentinel node employs a blue dye injected at the site of the tumor. It stains the sentinel node blue. The surgeon then makes a small incision in the lower axilla and looks for the blue dye in the lymphatic channels and the lymph node. The sentinel node is then removed and sent to a pathologist, who then examines it very carefully for evidence of any breast cancer cells. If the node is negative and has no evidence of cancer cells, then no further axillary dissection is needed. However, if the sentinel node does contain cancer cells and is positive, then a traditional axillary node dissection is recommended to determine if any other lymph nodes contain cancer.

The sentinel node dissection has been tested in several major medical centers. Its accuracy is very high and reliable, and it may soon become the standard of care for most breast cancer patients. If this technique is of interest to you, ask your surgeon about it.

■   ■   ■

## Lumpectomy, or Breast Conservation

Breast conservation, otherwise known as segmental mastectomy or lumpectomy or partial mastectomy, is the removal of only the tumor and a margin or border of normal tissue, and therefore only part of your breast. The malignant or cancerous tissue and a margin of healthy tissue (clean margins) are removed, along with some of the axillary nodes. Sometimes a quadrantectomy—removal of the quadrant (quarter or area) of breast in which the tumor is growing—will be recommended. This type of surgery is usually followed by a course of radiation therapy to treat the remainder of your breast.

Depending on how much tissue needs to be removed to achieve clean margins relative to the size of your breast, you may look more or less different than you did before the surgical procedures. Breast conservation may leave you completely satisfied with the cosmetic result, but be aware that some women are less happy with the outcome than others. If you feel truly unhappy with the appearance of your breast after all your treatment is over, it may be possible to undergo partial reconstruction. Talk with a plastic surgeon. Most women, however, decide over time that a less-than-perfect breast is a small price to pay for life.

## Mastectomy, or Breast Removal

There are two types of mastectomy surgery, and you may be presented with options.

- A simple (total) mastectomy (including the nipple/areola), in which all breast tissue, but nothing else, is removed
- A modified radical mastectomy, in which all breast tissue and some axillary lymph nodes are removed

Keep in mind that there are also variations on these options which your surgeon or oncologist might also describe to you. You may also be told that you can choose to have breast reconstruction, either at the same time you have a mastectomy or at a later date. You may decide to have a mastectomy and no other surgery. Many women find they adapt comfortably to life with a prosthesis, and for them, this is an entirely acceptable choice.

## Types of Reconstructive Surgery

Several types of reconstruction may be available to you. Following a mastectomy, reconstruction can be done either immediately (at the time of the mastectomy) or at a later date (many months or even years after). (There is usually no need for reconstruction after surgery less than mastectomy.) In either case, further procedures may be necessary in the months that follow—for example, placement of a nipple/areolar complex, reduction of the other side to match the reconstructed one, and so forth.

Reconstruction has become more common, but remember that you do have another option: mastectomy alone. In some hospitals immediate reconstruction is the standard of care, and women are told in the same breath that "you need to have a mastectomy, but you can have reconstruction at the same time." For many women, this may indeed be the best option, as they never have to deal with the total absence of a breast and do not have to make a decision to return in the future for more surgery. However, for others, this may be a mistake. You will find it hard to think clearly about these choices, some of which involve major surgery with long recoveries, while you are still trying to absorb the initial diagnosis of breast cancer. Remember that you can opt to take care of the cancer now, with a mastectomy, and then revisit the question of reconstruction next year or even five years from now.

Your plastic surgeon will likely tell you of his/her successes, and there most certainly are some. We have known women who have comfortably gone to nude beaches after breast reconstruction. However, you need to remember that not everyone is so happy with the result, and once a reconstruction is done, it is hard to undo. Talk with other women about their choices. Try to see several reconstructed breasts. Take a little time to consider your choices.

The technique of reconstruction may involve a saline implant, an expandable saline implant, a flap of tissue (muscle, fat, skin) moved from the abdomen (TRAM flap) or from the back (latissimus dorsi flap), and not infrequently both a flap and an implant. To determine which choice you prefer, you should do two things: first, schedule an appointment with one or more plastic surgeons to discuss your options; second, find women who have had the different procedures you are considering and talk to them. Although your plastic surgeon will be very knowledgeable about the various procedures, unless she has undergone the surgery herself, s/he will not know what it feels like to live with the results of the surgery on and inside the body ever after.

Occasionally, tissue expanders (temporary fillers to prepare your breast) are indicated; these are inserted during a series of procedures over several months. You will experience three stages of treatment. The first step will be the implanting of a tissue-expanding device that your surgeon will insert into your chest wall following the mastectomy itself. When you wake up from surgery, the device will already be in place. As the plastic surgeon will explain to you, s/he will expand your remaining tissue gradually over the next several months so as to accommodate an implant large enough to match the other side. This is accomplished by injecting saline solution through a porthole left exposed at the mastectomy site. After these expanding treatments are completed, s/he will schedule a time to both remove the expanding device and insert your permanent implant; this procedure will require that you return to the hospital.

Each of these reconstructive procedures involving tissue transfer is essentially a graft. You can expect to heal fairly rapidly after the first couple of days. The first twenty-four hours you will feel lousy; you have just had major surgery lasting several hours. You need time to recover from the effects of anesthesia as well as from the surgery itself. Try to cooperate with your nurse, who will urge you to turn, cough, and deep-breathe regularly, even though doing these things will hurt. Be aware that you will have odd-looking tubes hanging from your incisions; the tubes accumulate fluid (a mixture of blood and other body fluids) and will need to be emptied on a regular basis. When your surgeon determines that the drainage has slowed to an acceptable trickle, s/he will remove the tubes by exerting a steady, firm pressure at the site; the opening in the skin through which the tubes had been inserted will seal quickly (within one to two days).

You can expect to have some postoperative pain; however, you may be surprised that the mastectomy site itself is not the major source of discomfort. This is because the area is numb, following the severing of many nerves. The chest area will remain numb for weeks or months OR POSSIBLY FOREVER.

### Summary of Reconstruction Decisions

- There are both advantages and disadvantages to having simultaneous or immediate reconstruction.
- Advantages include having only one surgery, which also means one general anesthesia, one hospitalization, one recovery period, and not ever having to live without a breast.
- Disadvantages include having to make a complicated decision in the middle of a period of high anxiety and the small but real chance that the rest of your cancer treatment—for example, chemotherapy—might have to be delayed if there are unexpected surgical complications. It is best to begin chemotherapy when you have healed from your surgery. This is important because chemotherapy kills fast-growing cells and would impede your natural healing from surgery.
- Some women are very pleased with the cosmetic results of reconstruction. Others are not. It may be helpful to

think of your reconstructed breast as a "fashion accessory" rather than as a breast. It will not feel like a part of you for a long while. Anticipate an adjustment period of months or even years as you get used to this new body part, which will feel different both from the outside and on the inside. Be aware that a reconstructed breast following a mastectomy will neither have nor be able to register any sensation. It will be a permanently numb add-on.

## Post-Surgery

### Axillary Node Dissection

If you have had an axillary node dissection, you will experience discomfort under your arm and along the length of the arm, part of which may be numb while part may be sore. You may experience very brief but intense pain down the full length of your arm, even into your hand, for months. This is normal. You must use the affected arm as soon as you can and keep the arm elevated when you are sleeping or resting (remember those small pillows). Small pillows will help you support your sore arm and side more comfortably. If you don't own a couple of these, either buy them yourself before surgery or have someone get them for you. Your nurse or doctor may suggest that you see a physical therapist after the initial healing period; s/he will show you several exercises. You should do these exercises every day; neglecting to do them will impede your ability to recover range of motion—

for example, driving your car, lifting groceries or your children. Some women believe they are helped by massage therapy to feel more normal in the surgical area.

## Lymphedema

An annoying complication of axillary dissection (done either with mastectomy or lumpectomy) is lymphedema of the arm. Lymphedema is chronic swelling of the arm due to the accumulation of fluid as a result of lymph node surgery. This surgery can interfere with normal drainage. Lymphedema occurs very rarely following the limited type of axillary dissection usually done at the present time, but it does sometimes occur. Another temporary complication is limited motion of the shoulder. Normal activity right after surgery and active exercise ten to fourteen days later will alleviate this. If you find that you have limited use of your arm, ask for a referral to a physical therapist. If you have a problem, choose loose-fitting tops with deep, roomy armholes and be careful not to wear tight cuffs at the wrist or tight jewelry on that side. Try to avoid cuts or scrapes on the affected arm. Also be very careful about hangnails, paper cuts, and fissures in the cuticles. Be sure to apply a topical antiseptic and an adhesive bandage to speed healing. When you have a manicure, be sure to tell the manicurist to exercise extra caution. Wear gloves when you garden. Keep your hands moisturized. Seek medical attention immediately if you see signs or symptoms of an infection in that arm or hand (redness, pain, swelling, warmth). YOU WILL *ALWAYS* BE AT RISK FOR LYMPHEDEMA FOR ALL OF YOUR LIFE. THESE RULES APPLY NOW AND ALWAYS.

## Tips Post-Surgery

■ Vitamin E cream or the gel from vitamin E capsules may be applied on your scars as they start to heal. You could also try aloe vera (either pure gel or straight from the leaf of an aloe plant).

■ Be easy on yourself as you recover from surgery. Remember that you are healing both physically and emotionally.

■ If you have had reconstruction, your plastic surgeon will give you detailed instructions about what you can and cannot do. Anticipate many weeks of some restrictions on your physical activity.

■ If you have had a less major surgery, you will still have some limits imposed on your activity. Do not try to be a superwoman and do too much too soon. You will hurt yourself and slow down your recovery.

■ This is still the hardest time psychologically, and that difficulty is now compounded by the real physical changes you have experienced. You are well on your way to the time when it will seem a little easier, but do not expect to be there until you have made all of your treatment decisions and have embarked on whatever will come next.

■  ■  ■

# Nonsurgical Treatments

**Radiation Therapy**

Radiation therapy, following lumpectomy, is given five days a week for approximately six and a half weeks. The specific schedule of your treatment will be discussed with your radiation oncologist and nurse. If you are also getting chemotherapy, radiation may be administered at various points:

- Prior to chemotherapy
- Following chemotherapy
- "Sandwiched" in the middle of chemotherapy
- Concurrently with chemotherapy
- Recent studies have indicated the value of radiation for some women who have had mastectomies. If this is suggested to you, it will probably be at the end of your other treatments. You may have more trouble with skin burning when the radiation is directed at your chest wall rather than at a breast.

Most women find their radiation treatments to be relatively uneventful. It can be tiring to make a daily trip to the hospital, and it certainly is a daily reminder of what has happened to you. It may also require a major psychological shift to think of radiation as life-giving, instead of as an encounter to be avoided whenever possible.

In Hester's clinical practice, she has encountered some women who have a very difficult time psychologically during radiation therapy. Again, for most women, these treatments are quite manageable and sometimes more of an inconvenience than anything else. However, Hester believes that two groups of women may have real trouble during these weeks:

- Women who have a childhood history of sexual abuse
- Women whose primary coping mechanism is avoidance

Women in the first group may have a strong reaction to having to lie prone and still while a large and powerful object is suspended over them. These feelings may be intense but confusing, as they come from semiconscious or unconscious memory. If you know that you have a history of sexual abuse, it would be wise to talk over these feelings and your planned treatment with an experienced oncology social worker or other mental heath clinician. Unless you choose to do so, you do not need to tell your medical team of your history. You can simply say that this treatment is difficult for you and that, therefore, you will require a little extra time and attention.

Women who use avoidance as their coping mechanism have trouble with radiation because of its dailiness. Instead of coming to the hospital for a surgical procedure or chemotherapy treatment every few weeks, they will need to come every day. Thus there are daily reminders that this is really happening, that breast cancer has been diagnosed, and painful feelings are likely to erupt. If you find that you are feeling more frightened or sad during radiation, it will be helpful to talk about this either at a breast cancer support group (where you would be likely to find others who feel the same way) or with an oncology social worker.

You can start to take care of your skin as soon as your surgical wounds are healed. Starting before radiation begins may help you avoid skin problems. You may use *unscented* Lubriderm or 100% *Pure Aloe Gel* (the clear kind); both of these are widely available. After showering and at bedtime, apply to your whole breast and up to your armpit. Your radiation nurse will give you more information about skin care, acceptable soaps, and so forth. The basic theme is purity: Avoid using anything containing additives, fragrance, or metals on your affected skin. It is best to skip using deodorants (except fully natural ones) for the time being.

Before beginning radiation, you will have an appointment for radiation planning. This is a painless procedure, but one which many women find emotionally difficult because the environment is strange and the machines may seem quite intimidating. Ask questions if you wish. You will be asked to lie still, your hand up under your head and your breast/torso exposed, for approximately forty-five minutes while several people measure, mark, X-ray, and study the areas to be treated. Here are a few strategies that might help:

- You can bring a Walkman and listen to music.
- You can bring a companion to talk with.
- If you are still experiencing discomfort from your surgery when you raise your arm up above your head, take two Tylenol before you leave for the hospital.
- Marks (tattoos) will be put on your chest to guide the radiation. They are very small, but permanent. Rather

than what you imagine when you think "tattoo," these will be tiny pinprick-sized marks that are usually indistinguishable from freckles. You will feel the tattoo pinpricks, but the process is not painful.

■ It is theoretically possible to have these marks removed later by laser. Most radiation oncologists prefer that you not do this. If you should ever again require radiation therapy to this area, it would be extremely important to be able to exactly identify the area previously treated. The same place in your body usually can not be safely irradiated more than once (i.e., one series of treatments).

### Practical Tips for Radiation

■ Again, you may bring and listen to a Walkman.

■ You will spend time after undressing in a waiting room. Bathrobes are provided, but you may bring a jacket or wrap of your own. You can also wear a regular button-down-the-front blouse.

■ Talk with other women in the waiting room. You will see the same people there each day; lifelong friendships have been formed in this environment.

■ Consider bringing a friend. It can be a good time for a visit.

■ Let the technicians know if you like to chat or prefer silence.

■ Apply your moisturizer immediately after treatment and before you get dressed.

If you have moderate or worse burning on your skin (which is unlikely), ask your doctor if you can use goat's milk soap or Radia Care, a cream available at medical supply stores.

If you are using special creams or ointments on your skin, it may be helpful to wear a thin paper diaper liner between your breast and your bra to prevent stains on your clothing.

- Even if you generally take showers, try warm baths during radiation. They are very soothing.
- Cotton athletic bras and cotton camisoles are the most comfortable. There are pretty ones, and this is the time to splurge. Try searching through the natural fiber catalogs as well as the stores.
- Plan your daily radiation treatment as something you do on the way to somewhere else—not as the main event of your day.
- Parking may be a concern. Ask about places to park and the possibility of a reduced parking rate.

## Chemotherapy and Hormone Therapy

Many women will be given chemotherapy and/or hormone therapy as part of their treatment for breast cancer. Chemotherapy may be administered in conjunction with radiation or in sequence with radiation (either before or after) or independent of radiation treatments altogether. In most cases, chemotherapy is administered prophylactically or adjuvantly (to prevent a possible recurrence of the disease, not to treat known active cancer). Malignant breast tumors usually grow slowly over time, and in many cases, the tumors detected at the time the diagnosis is made have been growing for quite a while. Since some breast cancer cells have the ability to spread to other areas of the body (metastasize), chemotherapy or hormone therapy may be recommended to treat the disease systemically by killing any cells that may have traveled away from the primary tumor. When successful, this treatment will prevent recurrence of the disease.

Generally speaking, most breast cancers need to be treated both locally and systemically. Mastectomy or wide excision with radiation are the local treatment options; they are planned to prevent a recurrence of the cancer in your breast. They do nothing, however, to treat any cancer cells that may have already escaped the tumor and gone elsewhere in your body. Although your own immune system may be effective in destroying any traveling cells, the possibility that it may not be is the rationale for chemotherapy or hormone therapy. There is strong evidence from careful scientific studies that breast cancer is a systemic disease and that even in cases of women with negative axillary lymph nodes, there may already be cancer cells somewhere else.

The real danger of breast cancer is not what occurs in your breast but what potentially could happen in other parts of your body. If the breast cancer cells spread, or metastasize, to vital organs (for example, your lungs or your liver), it is a life-threatening situation.

Sometimes women wonder if they can safely avoid chemotherapy at the time of diagnosis, when it would be given adjuvantly, and receive the treatment only when/if the cancer recurs in the future. There is no easy way to say this. This is the time to do everything you possibly can to prevent any future recurrence of your breast cancer and to live a long and healthy life. Breast cancer that recurs in other parts of your body is treatable, but it is not usually curable. This first shot is your best shot at surviving breast cancer. Use it.

Chemotherapy for breast cancer is a changing science. As you talk with other women who were treated a few years ago, you will find that their regimens were somewhat different. There may also be differences of opinion among doctors and medical centers. Although this can seem frightening and confusing, it does not mean that one treatment is right and all the others are wrong. Conversely, research has shown that standard adjuvant chemotherapy treatments for breast cancer are *virtually* identical in outcome. You will make choices that reflect your personal needs.

Some adjuvant chemotherapy programs for breast cancer have been used for years and have proven their value over time. Clinical trials, carefully designed studies using different drugs or different schedules of treatment, are always in progress as doctors try to find even more effective ways to treat breast cancer. Slightly different treatment regimens are likely to be used in different parts of the country. All of them have the same goal: saving your life.

The most important thing is your health, now and in the future. You need to do what is best for you and what has the best chance of ensuring your long and healthy life. Remember that there is no single right choice of treatment. It is important that you receive appropriate chemotherapy, but there are likely to be several treatment regimens that are equally right for you.

Many women are more frightened by the prospect of chemotherapy than they were of surgery. It can be difficult to forget images you have seen in the movies or read in books of cancer patients being desperately ill from the chemotherapy treatments. Fortunately, times have changed and real progress has been made with controlling the nausea and vomiting you may be dreading. There are new and powerful drugs, such as Kytril and Zofran, which eliminate or greatly reduce these side effects. *Over time, there will be additional new drugs discovered and recommended as well.*

You may also be fearful of having such powerful drugs injected into your system. It can be hard to think of chemotherapy as lifesaving rather than as toxic poisons. Talk with your doctor about your concerns, and remember that a drug strong enough to kill cancer is going to be strong enough to have some other side effects. All of this is temporary. You are trying to save your life.

Talk with other women who have undergone chemotherapy about their experiences. What you hear from them will be somewhat different from what you hear from your doctors. Most women will tell you that their fantasies about chemotherapy were much worse than the reality. No one would suggest that receiving chemotherapy is pleasant, but it is completely manageable. Use all the information to help you make the best decision for yourself.

### Hormone Therapy

Tamoxifen is the most common hormonal therapy used for the systemic treatment of breast cancer. Tamoxifen has been used for many years to treat metastatic breast cancer, and more recently, to treat postmenopausal women with new breast cancer. Even more recently, it has been added to the full treatment of some younger women, usually after the completion of chemotherapy.

Breast cancers are classified as being either estrogen and progestrone receptor positive or negative. This will be one of the things described by the pathologist who reviews your tumor cells. Those cells which are er/pr positive require estrogen to grow and divide. Tamoxifen acts as an estrogen blocker (anti-estrogen), making any remaining cancer cells unable to respond to estrogen. The cells then die.

Many node-negative postmenopausal women whose breast cancers are er/pr positive will be given tamoxifen for five years in lieu of systemic chemotherapy. Older women whose breast cancers are er/pr negative may well receive chemotherapy. Occasionally, the situation demands that postmenopausal breast cancer be treated with both chemotherapy and tamoxifen.

Younger women whose tumors are er/pr positive may be advised to take tamoxifen, generally for a period of five years following their chemotherapy. Recent studies have indicated that the addition of tamoxifen to a woman's treatment may both reduce the risk of a recurrence of her existing breast cancer and reduce the risk of her developing a second (independent) breast cancer. Some oncologists are now recommending tamoxifen to their er/pr negative patients after chemotherapy. Ask him/her about this. A number of similar drugs are currently being studied, and soon there will likely be alternatives or additions to tamoxifen, some of which may have fewer undesirable side effects, such as enhanced risk of uterine cancer or pulmonary emboli.

Tamoxifen is taken orally, usually two small pills daily. If your doctor recommends tamoxifen to you, he/she will talk with you about the risks and benefits of this important drug. Taking tamoxifen may treat your cancer in the same way that taking chemotherapy would do, systemically, but the experience is not at all similar. The hardest part of tamoxifen for most women is remembering to take it.

When you are taking a medicine twice a day every day for five years, you may well find it hard to remember whether you have actually taken each dose. We have found it helpful to work out a system to remind you. If you take your medicine at your bathroom sink, try always putting the pill container on the left side of the sink in the morning and then, as soon as you take your morning dose, moving it to the right-hand side. This way, when evening comes and you see the container on the right side, you will know you took your dose that morning and can proceed to take that night's pill. Again, as soon as you swallow that night's pill, immediately move the container back to the left-hand side. Thus, if one morning you see that the container is still on the right side of the sink, you'll know you forgot to take your dose the previous evening. Do not assume you should take double doses; ask your own physician what s/he recommends you do about missed doses.

### Types of Chemotherapy

Several kinds of chemotherapy are frequently used to treat breast cancer. Your oncologist will speak to you about which drugs are most appropriate for your situation. Some of the common chemotherapy agents which have been used for years include Cytoxan, Adriamycin, Methotrexate, and 5-Fluorouracil (5-Fu). Others are being studied and used all the time, and it is likely that, over the next few years, standard chemotherapy combinations will be somewhat different than they are today. For example, Taxol or Taxotere are now sometimes added to adjuvant chemotherapy treatment. Usually the drugs are administered through an IV tube in your arm/hand and are not painful. It can be unsettling to realize that there is no standard treatment that is best for everyone, but you can be sure that your doctor is recommending what is best for you. Feel free to ask questions, and, if you wish, to get a second opinion.

The prospect of undergoing chemotherapy is frightening. Many women are more worried about chemotherapy than surgery. Start by forgetting all the horror stories you have heard. Remember that each person reacts as an individual to treatment; it is also crucial that you realize your oncologist wants to help minimize any unpleasant side effects you may experience. However, s/he can only do so if you communicate how you are feeling; physicians cannot read minds. Your oncology nurse will become a person upon whom you will rely heavily; s/he will help prepare you for your treatments by talking with you, providing you with booklets and information sheets, and answering questions you will have. Remember to communicate how you are feeling; *if you need help, ask for it*. Don't assume that if you feel very ill, you must suffer in silence; while some discomfort is to be expected, many medicines and salves may provide you with relief. You should not be miserable from chemotherapy! Call your doctor if you are. *There is no correlation between how "ill" you become from chemotherapy and whether you derive benefit from it.*

Many people are surprised to find that while chemotherapy is not a pleasant experience, it is actually bearable. You can go about your usual business, although you may wish to alter your work schedule slightly if that is an option for you. It is a rare supervisor or boss who would not be sympathetic to your request during the months you are on treatment.

Some women have jobs that they find too difficult to manage during chemotherapy. If this is true for you, inquire about short-term disability, extended sick leave, or sick day banks. There is likely to be something that will help you financially if you decide to take a leave from work.

If you can possibly arrange to have a family member or close friend accompany you to your chemotherapy sessions, do so. Ask someone who has a calming, soothing effect on you; you need support and encouragement at this time, not additional anxiety or escalating fear. Depending on the time of day you schedule your treatments and whether you will be returning home or going on to work, you may want to have someone come with you who will also be able to drive you to the hospital and back home again. After your first treatment, you may decide that you want company for all your treatments, or you may decide you are more comfortable going alone. If possible, try to arrange to have someone go with you the first time. It will be helpful to have a companion who can support and distract you; you may also be very glad to have someone else contend with driving and parking.

Most people feel okay for several hours following chemotherapy treatments; they are able to eat, work, do errands, and so forth. Usually some reaction occurs four to six hours later; there are some people who experience little reaction until twenty-four or even forty-eight hours later. On the other hand, some people feel the worst twelve or twenty-four hours following treatment. You will have to see how you feel.

Expect that the first treatment will be a new experience both for you and also for those caring for you. If it goes well, the odds are good that the remaining treatments will, too. Your oncologist may decide to change or adjust the dosage or the anti-nausea medications depending on your reactions following treatment. You may or may not experience a variety of side effects; if you want to know what to expect, ask your oncologist or your chemo nurse to tell you about these. Realize that you personally may experience some, none, or all of the possible side effects. Realize, too, that each treatment cycle may be different.

### Side Effects

*Nausea and Fatigue.* There are many anti-nausea medications available; your physician and chemo nurse will work together with you to find out what works best for you. Modern pharmacology can go a long way toward alleviating, or at least minimizing, your physical reactions. There are three points at which you are likely to experience nausea: shortly after receiving IV chemotherapy, and/or twenty-four or forty-eight hours following the IV, and during the time you take Cytoxan pills (fourteen days of each month/cycle). The first problem can be helped by anti-emetic medication. The second problem, which may or may not happen to you, is comparable to morning sickness during pregnancy; this may slow you down, but will not incapacitate you or force you to radically curtail your normal activities. You may experience fatigue on and off over the course of each cycle. This will not be debilitating fatigue, and you will find that with some modification of your routine and your sleep schedule, you can manage to keep going.

The desired anti-cancer effects of chemotherapy are in no way directly related to the presence, absence, or intensity of side effects. The putative relationship is a kind of old wives' tale that springs from the same source as the stories that frighten women unnecessarily about side effects during pregnancy—for example, if you are not violently ill with morning sickness, then something must be wrong with your baby. Here are some suggestions for handling side effects:

- Eat a light meal before coming for chemotherapy.
- Chinese food the night before chemotherapy may help if you have difficult veins. Another strategy is to drink lots of fluids for twenty-four hours before a treatment.
- Nibble on something that appeals to you; an empty stomach will not help. Although many women report that they don't necessarily feel better if they eat something, everyone finds that she feels worse if she doesn't have anything in her stomach.
- Comfort foods may help. We've heard of preferences for everything from chicken soup to egg salad and hot dogs with mustard. Starches and carbohydrates may go down more easily; try bread, rice, potatoes, or puddings.
- Try not to skip breakfast. An empty stomach will exacerbate all symptoms.

- Try oatmeal or other hot cereals; think in terms of coating and settling your stomach.
- Experiment with mint, chamomile, or other herb teas.
- Try cinnamon or mint sugarless chewing gum.
- The combination of hot chocolate and peppermint candies may help.
- A very effective anti-nausea concoction is a mixture of equal parts of lemon juice and fresh ginger with sugar and salt added to taste. Take a spoonful or add it to a beverage.
- If you're taking Cytoxan pills, experiment with varying the time of day you take them.
- Your doctor may advise you not to take the Cytoxan pills at night, but otherwise you can take them after each meal, in between meals, all together after one meal, or in any other combination you choose.
- If you're taking Cytoxan pills, you may want to enlist someone else's help (a friend or your child if s/he is old enough) by asking him or her to suggest a guided imagery when you are about to take your pills. They might verbalize suggestions such as "Imagine you are picking up a mint or candy; feel the smooth coating on your tongue," and so forth.
- If you are taking Cytoxan pills, try not to look at them. Ask someone else to hand them to you.
- Alternative techniques such as meditation, relaxation, acupuncture, or hypnosis may help you. If these techniques appeal to you, investigate them.
- Constipation is a frequent side effect of some anti-nausea medications. Start taking a stool softener, like Senokot or Senokot-S, two days before your chemotherapy treatment.

■ Mouth sores can be a very unpleasant side effect of some chemotherapy drugs. If you are receiving a drug that is likely to cause mouth sores, your doctor or nurse will give you a mouthwash such as Peridex. Start to use it at the first sign of mouth sores!

Many women find that fatigue during chemotherapy is a bigger problem than nausea. Here are some suggestions for taking care of yourself and managing fatigue:

■ This is not a time to push yourself to stay up late or get up early. Try to get at least eight hours of sleep at night. You may well find that you need ten or more hours to feel rested.

■ Sticking with a bedtime routine may help you fall asleep. Try a warm bath, reading in bed, or something hot to drink.

■ Even when you feel exhausted, it can be hard to sleep through the night because your mind is so active. Most women find themselves, in the early days of breast cancer, awakening at 2:00 A.M., and starting to worry about all the things that might happen. If you are awake and frightened or sad, awaken your partner for a short talk or hug. Write your worries down and tell yourself you will deal with them in the morning. Try meditation or listening to soothing music.

■ Many women ask their doctors for a sleep medication during breast cancer treatment. This is often a good idea and you will be able to stop taking it later.

■ When you are feeling exhausted and short of energy, try

to prioritize your tasks. Do first what is most important.

- What jobs can you ask or hire someone else to do? For example, if the laundry feels overwhelming, there are laundromats where you can drop off your dirty clothes and pick them up clean and folded.
- Explore home delivery services of groceries, dry cleaning, laundry, etc.
- Take short naps as you need them.

*Hair Loss.* Many women find that losing their hair from chemotherapy is the most disturbing thing that happens. (Talk with your oncologist about what to expect from your chemotherapy. Not all the drugs used cause the same degree of hair loss.) You should go to see someone who sells wigs while you still have your own hair so that there will be the best chance for a good match of color, texture, and style. Of course you may decide that you want to deal with hair loss by using hats, scarves, turbans, or a combination of all of these. Even when you are told that hair loss may or is likely to happen to you, it is still traumatic. Since this may begin to happen within the first three weeks of treatment, you will want to think about this as soon as you can. If you have a close friend or family member who can go with you to look at wigs, plan to go with her. As you decide on the type of wig to purchase, bear in mind that a synthetic or mixed fiber wig is not only less expensive but is also lighter, cooler, and more comfortable to wear.

Your doctor or nurse can give you an accurate guess as to when you might lose your hair. It is very predictable and depends on what chemotherapy drugs you are receiving. Some women find that their scalp becomes quite sore or tender a few days before the hair loss begins. This may not happen to you, but if it does, consider it a forty-eight-hour warning.

There is no way to make the actual experience of losing your hair anything less than a crisis. As hard as this is to imagine, it will be easier to bear once the hair is gone. The anticipation of the loss and the actual process of losing it are the worst. One strategy for when your hair begins to go is often very helpful for many people. You will know with certainty when this is happening; if you are wondering whether your hair is coming out, it is not. If you can muster the courage and determination to do so, consider having your hair buzzed and/or your head shaved. Many women find that their hairdresser is more than willing to meet them before or after hours at the salon or even to come to their home to do this. Your husband/friend/partner could also provide this service to you. Taking it off, all of it, puts you in control and gets you through it as quickly as possible. Once the hair is gone, you will start to adjust to your new bald head.

One woman whose hair came out in the early spring was enormously helped by her husband's tender suggestion of putting clumps of hair in and near the bushes and trees in their yard. He said that birds would use the hair to build their nests, and this turned out to be true. In the fall, when the leaves were gone and the nests visible, she found several empty nests warmly and softly lined with her hair.

Here are some additional practical tips for hair loss:

- Buy a small metal screening device (available at a hardware store) that you put over your shower drain to prevent the large quantities of hair from blocking your drain.

- Keep an empty plastic bowl in the shower to collect the hair as it comes out.
- Adjust the water volume on the showerhead to protect your scalp, which may become quite sensitive.
- A satin pillowcase may be more comfortable on a tender scalp.
- You can put a linen tea towel over your pillow to facilitate morning cleanup while you are shedding. Some people like to wear a disposable cap (the kind cafeteria workers use) to bed.
- Be aware that you may experience additional hair loss elsewhere or everywhere on your body; this may include eyebrows and eyelashes, as well as body hair.
- Stop by a cosmetics counter in a department store. Ask about using powdered eye shadow to draw eyebrows.
- You may wish to join a "Look Good . . . Feel Better" program, which is designed to assist women undergoing cancer treatment. See the resources section or ask.
- When your treatments are completed and your hair begins to grow in, you may be able to speed up the process if you take brewer's yeast or wheat grass tablets and massage your scalp with conditioner.

Sometimes hair begins to grow back before the end of chemotherapy. This does *not* mean that the drugs are not working! It is just more evidence that everyone is different. As your hair grows in, it will probably be curly (even if you have always had straight hair). It may straighten out as it gets longer and the weight pulls it down, or you may have wavy or curly hair for the rest of your life. The color, too, may be different—obviously you may have more gray than you remember, but some women report different shades of brown or blond. Consider other coloring options, too. You may decide to dye your hair a new shade you have never tried before. Or you may wish to experiment with a different hairstyle and color as you reconsider your new self-image. Consider this time an opportunity for refashioning yourself.

Here are some tips for appropriate headgear:

- *Big* works best! Scarves should be at least forty inches square. In spite of what you may be told, there is no such thing as too big.
- Rayon is the fabric of choice. It clings to itself, drapes nicely, can be washed. Cotton is a good second option.
- Silk scarves are lovely second layers but slip right off bald heads!
- Fringed scarves can be used very successfully, and the movement of the fringe is reminiscent of hair.
- Look in fabric stores for material to use as scarves; you may find greater choice and many more bargains than in department stores. Buying fabric is cheaper than buying scarves. Don't bother to hem the pieces; simply tuck the edges in.
- A soft cotton baby diaper can be worn under a scarf to increase the height and achieve a different look.
- Check out the scarf selection, too, at stores selling clothing from India or other import shops.
- Remember the possibilities of layering. Use a solid-color rayon scarf as the first layer, then top it with a print silk or cotton scarf twisted into a rope and wound around

your head. Or top the bottom layer with an attractive, colorful man's tie, a fabric belt, ribbons, or a hat over a scarf.

- Try putting pretty pins on your scarf or turban.
- Cotton bandannas can be sewn together to make informal, inexpensive (and big enough) colorful scarves.
- This is the moment to experiment with big earrings and maybe a bit more lip color and makeup than usual.

# notes

notes

# chemically induced *menopause*

**Very often the** drugs administered during chemotherapy will cause the suspension of your monthly periods. During chemotherapy, if your periods continue, they are very likely to be different from your usual periods in duration and flow. Some women experience an increase in flow, accompanied by fairly heavy cramping, during the first month or two; other women notice a decrease in flow that precedes cessation. Depending on your age and how close you are to naturally occurring menopause, your menstrual cycle may resume or it may not. Although there has been a great deal of attention directed to the experience of passing through menopause, you may find, as many of us did, that when you are coping with cancer, menopause pales in comparison; it is simply not that big a deal.

Yet, in spite of the understanding that being alive is much more important than unexpectedly having an early menopause, it is also true that some of us really hate it. Women who have not completed their families may have the most painful adjustment. Even if they would have decided not to have (more) children, having the choice taken away can be devastating. We often feel out of control and victimized or "done to" because of the cancer, and this can be one more significant example of what we have lost.

## Side Effects: Sexuality and Hot Flashes

The two side effects that are most difficult are hot flashes and the changes in sexuality. The frequency, intensity, and duration of hot flashes vary a lot from person to person. Some of us have only an occasional "warm flash," while others of us drip with sweat. It is impossible to predict how many, how bad, and how long. You will become accustomed to your own rhythms of hot flashes, and you will find some strategies that help. They seem to be worse at night, at times of stress, and when the temperature is high. If you don't already have air-conditioning in your bedroom, this might be a time to consider buying a unit.

The sexual side effects of menopause are also variable. The two general areas of change are in libido and vaginal dryness or elasticity. It is easy to blame these changes on the sudden loss of estrogen, and that, no doubt, is a big part of the problem. There are other contributing factors unique to women going through breast cancer. It is hard to feel sexy and desirable when you are bald, tired, and perhaps nauseated. The blows to your self-image and sense of womanliness are strong. Some women also feel assaulted by the many medical exams, all of which seem to involve breast exams. As much as you may love your partner, there may be times when you just do not want anyone else to touch you.

Changes in libido can happen suddenly or gradually. You may find that you have difficulty reaching orgasm or even that the previously erogenous zones of your body seem to have turned to wood. The same stroking or touching that used to feel wonderful may feel like nothing. In Hester's groups, women are relieved to learn that they are not alone with these feelings. It is ironic that at a time when you may long for closeness and emotional comforting, you are uninterested in sex. The best way to manage is to talk honestly with your partner about what you are or are not feeling, reassure him or her that this is not about love and that it likely will get better in time. Most women have a slow and gradual improvement in response after treatment ends. The unfortunate truth is that you may never be quite as sexually sensitive as you were before. We hope, if that is the case, that the enrichment of your emotional relationships by virtue of what you are going through may provide some compensation. Many couples find that their love for each other is enhanced in ways never before imagined.

# Practical Tips
# for Symptoms of Menopause

- Because you have had breast cancer, you probably cannot take estrogens. Currently there are clinical trials underway to determine the safety of HRT (hormone replacement therapy) for women who have had breast cancer. You may want to talk with your doctor about this in the future. There are other strategies for dealing with menopausal symptoms. Find a gynecologist who is experienced with women who have had breast cancer.

- Some women find that hot flashes are helped by eating soy products or drinking soy milk or taking vitamin E (800 units a day). Look carefully at any holistic menopause treatments: many contain natural or plant estrogens. *Before taking them, be sure to consult your physician.*

- A few prescription medicines you can safely take may help. Ask your doctor about the clonidine patch (otherwise known as a blood pressure medicine), bellemene s, or about a low dose of Effexor.

- Remember the handheld fans which your mother or grandmother used. They are still available (look in Asian markets), and they still work.

- Hot flashes tend to be worse at times of stress—another good reason to try to reduce the stress in your life.

- Dress in layers. Try V-neck shirts or blouses with a cardigan-style sweater or jacket over them for warmth. The outer layers can then be removed when the flash strikes. Scoop-neck or jewel-neck tops make an excellent choice for a first layer, too. You will probably want to avoid turtlenecks at this time.

- If you have hot flashes at night, keep an extra pillow near you. When you awaken in a sweat, switch to the fresh, cool pillow. It helps. Also, keep fresh drinking water next to your bed along with a few mints or suckers.

- One woman who had many intense night sweats kept a small cooler by her bed. During the day, she left two or three wet washcloths in the freezer and put them by her bed at night.

- There are good over-the-counter products to alleviate vaginal dryness. It makes sense to try several brands to see what works best for you. Astroglide is a frequent favorite. It may be helpful to use a product like Replens every other day as you begin chemotherapy to minimize vaginal dryness. You can also use plain yogurt as a lubricant for intercourse.

- Like lots of things in life, the old cliché of "use it or lose it" applies here.

- A vitamin E capsule opened and spread on the vagina increases vaginal lubrication.

- There is some research suggesting that the topical vaginal use of Retin-A may help with dryness and elasticity. Ask your gynecologist.

- When your treatments are completed, if you are experiencing chronic difficulties with your libido, ask your oncologist about the possibility of taking a low dose of testosterone.

- Remember Kegel exercises? These are still one of the best ways to strengthen your pelvic floor and enhance sexual sensation. The easiest way to practice these exercises is during urination. As you begin to pee, squeeze your muscles together to stop the flow. Stop and start it several times. After doing this a few times, you will have identified the correct muscles to contract and can then practice at other times. When you do so, contract the muscles and hold them for a slow count of ten; then relax.

- Expect some changes in your sex life. Be willing to adapt.
- Your sexual interest and response will probably return to normal after your treatments end.
- If this doesn't happen, be creative and find other, new ways of both receiving and giving physical pleasure.
- Make up your mind to deal with your cancer. Be determined to get through it.
- Know that you will need to face painful and difficult changes, including an altered image of yourself, both physically and emotionally.
- Allow yourself to grieve for these losses—of full health, of body parts, and of your former self. Never again will you feel carefree in the same innocent way.
- Be good to yourself.
- Try to see the humorous side of life. Rent funny movies.
- Enjoy what you do and do what you enjoy.
- Tell people who ask what you need. They want to help you.
- Learn to both ask for help and accept it.
- Be kind to yourself and remember to laugh often.
- Let yourself cry.
- There is light at the end of the tunnel!
- YOU *CAN* DO THIS. YOU ARE NOT ALONE.

# notes

notes

# survivorship *issues*

**Having breast cancer** will change you. With luck and the safe passage of time, you will find ways to appreciate what this life-changing diagnosis has done for you. You will grieve for the woman you used to be as you come to understand and value the woman you are becoming. The process you will pass through is complex and multifaceted and will demand your energy, your attention, and all of your patience. It is a journey in much the same way that life itself is. The final destination for everyone is, of course, death. But if you continually focus only on the destination, you will miss the journey, and it is the process of living day by day, and night by night, that constitutes the voyage. The final destination will come soon enough.

Living with breast cancer is similar in many ways to grieving other losses. As those of you who have suffered the loss of a dear one or other life tragedies already know, grieving is a complex and demanding task. It takes patience and courage. You will find, as time passes, that you experience a wide range of feelings and reactions. Some common feelings include:

- Shock, disbelief, denial, and anger
- Active suffering in the mourning process, letting the pain penetrate and register, letting yourself feel and express joy and sorrow
- Acceptance (and this happens only slowly)—coming to peace with yourself, your altered image, the loss of your former state of health and your sense of immortality, perhaps the loss of body parts and perhaps the loss of the potential to conceive and bear a child. You have lost who you were and will grow into who you will be.

Most, if not all of us, have confronted serious challenges and threats in our lives before being diagnosed with cancer. We did our best to address these situations, work through them, and then put them behind us as we moved on with our lives. In fact, this strategy is fully applicable to many kinds of cancer, since once the patient has passed the five-year mark, she can usually be pronounced cured. Unfortunately, the same cannot be said with certainty about breast cancer. While it is true that with every year that passes, it is more likely that breast cancer will be a part of our past, this is not always the case. The disease has been known to recur five, ten, fifteen, and even twenty years later. Thus, living with breast cancer becomes a particularly stressful challenge. Hester described the challenge well in a letter she wrote to the editor of our local newspaper. "All of life must be viewed through a double lens, that of possible future good health and that of possible future disaster.

Learning to live well after breast cancer is a lesson in hope."

Once you get through this ordeal, each of you will find your own way of beginning the next part of your life, choosing your own path, marking your own priorities. One thing is certain, whatever decisions you may choose: You will make changes in your life. Having cancer forces you to assess and reassess what you want to do with the rest of your life. If there are projects you have fantasized about but have pushed out of your consciousness, you may well decide to take the plunge and go ahead. This book is one of our projects.

The challenge is to learn how to live well, whatever that means to you personally. Although the terror you feel now, at the time of diagnosis, will subside and lose its intensity, it will remain a lifelong companion. Your awareness of it will, of course, fluctuate, and some days you will struggle not to be overwhelmed by it, while other days you will feel calmer and more in control. The overarching goal is to keep trying to achieve a balance in our lives between fear and hope. Whether healthy and well, or ill and unwell, we struggle to find level ground—a safe place where we feel the various competing attentions in our lives are in equilibrium.

We know that our shared goal must be to learn to live *as though* our cancer will never come back. Surely if we spend our lives struggling with fear and grief, the cancer has won—whether or not it ever recurs. If this is a challenge you must face in the future, you will find a way to do so. There will be moments and days when you are sad and afraid. Accept them. Know that sometimes, for all of us, the fear is like a wildcat on our backs, claws digging in. Try not to let it contaminate your joy and your appreciation for life. Instead, work toward seeing and appreciating how fragile and how wonderful life is!

Because we are all human, all of us must live with our own mortality. Birth and death are the two ultimate moments that define our lives. Our most gifted artists and poets have expressed the human condition in these terms since the beginning of recorded time.

We want to conclude by wishing you well on your journey and would like to leave two very different images with you, images that capture the two polarities between which we have often found ourselves vacillating: deep fear and exultant expectation. The first was written by the seventeenth-century British poet Andrew Marvell. Using a compelling image, Marvell describes forcefully the pressure of time that we who have been diagnosed with a life-threatening illness feel so acutely. The second image is contained within a poem written about two hundred years later by the American poet Emily Dickinson. Dickinson expresses beautifully the uplifting, energizing quality of keeping hope alive within. In the challenging weeks and months ahead of you, we encourage you to find your own balance.

> But at my back I always hear
> Time's winged charriot hurrying near.
> > —ANDREW MARVELL (1621–1678)

> "Hope" is the thing with feathers—
> That perches in the soul—
> And sings the tune without the words—
> And never stops—at all—
> > —EMILY DICKINSON (1830–1886)

# notes

notes

*resources*

## Support Groups

We believe that support groups are the very best resource for many of us. To locate a group near you:

- Ask your doctors or nurses for suggestions.
- Ask if there is an oncology social worker at your hospital. Ask her or him.
- Call the social work department of a nearby hospital and ask.
- Look in the community events section of your local newspaper.
- Call the local office of the American Cancer Society.
- Call the National Alliance of Breast Cancer Organizations at 212-719-0154.
- Call the National Cancer Institute's Cancer Information Service at 800-4-CANCER and ask for the names of certified mammography programs in your area. Call them.

# National Breast Cancer Organizations

- The American Cancer Society has a toll-free hotline, printed information about all kinds of cancer, and many service programs (e.g., Reach to Recovery, Road to Recovery) that are available locally. Look for the number of the nearest office to you in the white pages of your telephone book or call the national headquarters for their location. ACS, 1599 Clifton Road NE, Atlanta, GA 30329; 404-320-3333 or 800-ACS-2345

- The Komen Alliance is a comprehensive program for information, research, and support of breast cancer. The Susan G. Komen Foundation, Occidental Tower, 5005 LBJ Freeway, Suite 370, Dallas, TX 75224; 214-450-1777 or 800-I'M AWARE

- National Alliance of Breast Cancer Organizations (NABCO) is a national central resource center about breast cancer. They have a very complete resource list, a quarterly newsletter, customized information packets, and special mailings. NABCO, 9 East 37th St., 10th fl, New York, NY 10016; 212-719-0154

- National Breast Cancer Coalition was formed in 1991 as an advocacy and policy organization to involve women with breast cancer and their supporters in efforts to change public policy. There are also many state and local member organizations that share the goals of influencing breast cancer research funding and access to screening and clinical trials. NBCC, 1707 L

Street NW, Suite 1060, Washington, DC 20036; 202-296-7477

- National Coalition for Cancer Survivorship is a national network of groups concerned with issues of cancer survivorship for patients and their families. NCCS, 1010 Wayne Avenue, 5th floor, Silver Spring, MD 20910, 301-650-8868
- The Wellness Community has wonderful and extensive support and educational programs for cancer patients and their families at their many offices around the country. All services are free. Call the national headquarters to locate the Wellness Community nearest to you. TWC, 2716 Ocean Park Boulevard, Suite 1040, Santa Monica, CA 90405; 310-314-2555
- Y-ME National Breast Cancer Organization provides support, counseling, and connections to other women through their national toll-free hotline. There is also a hotline for partners. Y-ME, 212 W. Van Buren Street, Chicago, IL 60607; 312-986-8228 or 800-221-2141
- YWCA of the U.S.A.'s Encore Plus Program provides early detection, outreach, education, and exercise programs for women in YWCAs nationally. YWCA, 202-628-3636

## Cancer Hotlines and Information Numbers

- American Cancer Society's toll-free hotline provides information and referrals. 800-ACS-2345

- AMC Cancer Research Center's Cancer Information Line with counselors who can answer questions, provide support, and send information. Open Monday through Friday, 8:30–5:00 MST. 800-525-3777
- Cancer information service of the National Cancer Institute gives information and referrals. 800-4-CANCER
- Chemocare is a national agency that matches individual cancer patients with another who has the same problem. 800-55-CHEMO or 908-233-1103 in New Jersey.
- National Self Help Clearing House can refer you to local self-help services, especially regarding insurance and employment issues. 212-642-2944.
- Y-ME Breast Cancer Hotline offers support, referrals, and connections to other women. 800-221-2141

**Look Good . . . Feel Better**

This is a national beauty-focused program designed specifically for women undergoing chemotherapy or radiation treatments. It is sponsored by the Cosmetic, Toiletry, and Fragrance Association Foundation in partnership with the American Cancer Society and the National Cosmetology Association. You can find the most convenient location by calling your local American Cancer Society.

# Specialized Resources

- American Academy of Medical Acupuncture provides a referral line of medical doctors who practice acupuncture. AAMA, 5820 Wilshire Blvd, Suite 500, Los Angeles, CA 90036; 800-521-2262

- American Association of Naturopathic Physicians publishes a directory of their members. AANP, 601 Valley Street, Suite 105, Seattle, WA 98102; 206-298-0126

- American Association of Oriental Medicine can provide names of certified acupuncturists. AAOP, 433 Front Street, Catasauga, PA 18032; 610-266-1433

- American Holistic Medical Association publishes a directory. AHMA, 6728, Old Mclean Village Drive, Mclean, VA 22101; 703-556-9728

- American Institute for Cancer Research provides information on cancer and nutrition. To order written materials, write to AICR, 1759 R St., Washington, DC 20009. They also offer a nutrition-related hotline at 800-843-8114.

- American Massage Therapy Association can make referrals to a massage therapist in your area. Massage can be a terrific stress reducer and a wonderfully therapeutic boon! Try to include this in your high priority list of budgeted items. AMTA, 820 Davis St., Suite 100, Evanston, IL 60201; 847-864-0123 website: www.amtamassage.org

- Association of Oncology Social Work can make referrals to an oncology social worker in your area. AOSW, 1910 E. Jefferson St., Baltimore, MD 21205; 410-614-3990

- BMT Newsletter is a bimonthly newsletter for people considering or who have undergone bone marrow transplants. 1985 Spruce Ave. Highland Park, IL 60035; 708-831-1913

- *Coping Magazine* is a national publication for cancer patients. Media America, 2019 North Carothers, Franklin, TN 37064; 615-790-2400
- Lesbian Community Cancer Project, 4753 North Broadway, Suite 602, Chicago, IL 60640; 773-561-4662
- Living Beyond Breast Cancer, 111 Forrest Avenue, Narberth, PA 18072; 610-668-1320; website: www.lbbc.org
- MAMM is a new national magazine devoted to issues of women's cancers. MAMM, 349 West 12th Street, New York, NY 10014, 888-901-6266
- Mautner Project for Lesbians with Cancer, 1707 I Street NW, Suite 500, Washington, DC 20036; 202-332-5536
- National Black Women's Health Project, 1211 Connecticut Avenue, NW Suite 310, Washington, DC 20036; 202-835-0117
- National Bone Marrow Transplant Link is an information clearing house on bone marrow transplants. 29209 Northwestern Hwy 624, Southfield, MI 48034; 810-932-8483 or 800-LINK-BMT
- National Lymphedema Network provides both patients and professionals with information about prevention and treatment of lymphedema. 2211 Post St., Suite 404, San Francisco, CA 94115; 800-541-3259
- National Insurance Consumer Hotline can answer questions; 800-942-4242
- Office of Alternative Medicine at the National Cancer Institute can provide information about complementary therapies. OAM, 31 Center St., Bldg. 31, Room 5b38, Bethesda, MD 20892; 888-644-6226

■   ■   ■

# Internet Sites

There are many Internet sites with information about breast cancer. It is impossible to provide a complete list, but most of these sites will also have links to others. Remember to carefully evaluate what you read on the Web; you can find lots of opinions and some are not backed up with sound facts. Be careful about breast cancer chat rooms; they may be overwhelming and frightening at this time.

Association of Cancer Online Resources
   http://www.acor.org

Stanford Community Breast Health Project
   http://www-med.stanford.edu

American Cancer Society's Breast Cancer Site
   http://www.cancer.org/bcn.html

Avon Breast Cancer Crusade
   http://www.avon.com/about/awareness/frame.html

Breast Cancer Awareness: Two Sisters' Stories
   http://www.azstarnet.com/~pud

Cancer Care (Also in Spanish)
   http://www.cancercareinc.org

CancerNet Web Contents
   http://biomed.nus.sg//Cancer/contents.html

Cancer News, A Publication
   http://www.cancernews.com

Oncolink (Breast Cancer)
   http://cancer.med.upenn.edu/disease/breast

National Breast Cancer Coalition
   http://www.natlbcc.org

Onhealth.com
   http://www.onhealth.com

Mothers Supporting Daughters with Breast Cancer
http://www.azstarnet.com/~pud/msdbc/index.html

My Web md.com
http://www.mywebmd.com

Kidscope to Help Parents
http://www.kidscope.org

Breast Cancer Net
http://www.breastcancer.net

National Cancer Institute
http://www.nci.nih.gov

National Cancer Institute's Clinical Trials Site
http://cancertrials.nci.nih.gov

Information re Reconstruction
http://phudson.com/breastrec.html

Y-Me Has a Page for Kids
http://www.y-me.org

# Guided Imagery/Stress Release Tapes

Most cities will have audiotapes available in New Age book-stores, health food stores, and some regular music stores. Tapes are also available on the Web; remember Amazon.com and other book/music stores on the Internet.

Some stores carrying such tapes provide headsets at the store so you can listen before you purchase. This is especially helpful because your reaction to the sound of another person's voice is simply a matter of individual taste. Your favorite music may turn out to be the most soothing.

Lastly, we suggest getting tapes of varying lengths. You might want a 45-minute tape at the end of the workday to unwind, but a 10- or 20-minute pick-me-up might be more realistic in the middle of the day.

1. Emmett Miller, M.D.
   *Letting Go of Stress*
   *Ten-Minute Stress Manager*
   *Healing Journey*
   A catalog of tapes and an order form can be obtained from:
   SOURCE
   P.O. Box W
   Stanford, CA 94309
   1-800-52-TAPES

2. Mary Richards
   *High Mountain Meditation*
   *New Day's Promise*
   *Sunset on the Bay*
   A brochure can be obtained from:
   Master Your Mind
   881 Hawthorne Drive
   Walnut Creek, CA 94596
   510-945-0941

3. Robert Gass, Ph.D.
   *On Wings of Song*
   A catalog can be obtained from:
   Spring Hill Music
   P.O. Box 800
   Boulder, CO 80306

4. Belle Ruth Naparstek
   "Staying Well with Guided Imagery"
   800-800-8661

5. Bernie Siegel, M.D.
   *Meditation for Everyday Living*
   Tapes available through:
   Creative Audio
   Department BSS
   8751 Osborne
   Highland, IN 46322
   or
   ABC Audiovisual Enterprises, Inc.
   Department BSS
   500 West End Avenue #5B
   New York, NY 10024

## One: Introduction

**12**  David Spiegel, Joan R. Bloom, Helena Kraemer, and Ellen Gottheil, "Effect of Psychosocial Treatment on Survival of Patients with Metastatic Breast Cancer," *The Lancet*, October 14, 1989, 888–891.

## Two: Gathering Information/ Choosing Your Team

**29**  Miriam Wetzel, David Eisenberg, and Ted Kaptchuk, "Courses Involving Complementary and Alternative Medicine at U.S. Medical Schools," *Journal of the American Medical Association* 280 (9): 784–87.

# bibliography

There are many excellent books about breast cancer. A search on the Internet of Amazon.com lists 750 titles on this subject. These are some we can recommend; please let us know if you have other favorites.

Alpha Institute. *The Alpha Book on Cancer and Living*. Alpha Institute, Alameda, CA, 1993.

*A most comprehensive guidebook.*

*Art.Rage.Us: Art and Writing by Women with Breast Cancer*. With an introduction by Jill Eikenberry and epilogue by Terry Tempest Williams. Chronicle Books, San Francisco, 1998.

Austin, Steve, and Cathy Hitchcock. *Breast Cancer: What You Should Know (And May Not Be Told) About Prevention, Diagnosis, and Treatment*. Prima Publishing, Rocklin, CA, 1994.

*A husband-and-wife team, the authors walk you through each part of diagnosis and treatment (both conventional and alternative) and prevention*

Bailis, Kathryn. "College Age Daughters of Women with Breast Cancer: How They Cope," unpublished manuscript submitted at Colgate University, Hamilton, NY, December 1996. For more information contact bailis@nobles.edu or call 617-484-0386 or fax 617-489-2484.

Blumberg, Rena. *Headstrong*. Crown Publishers, Inc., New York, 1982.

Brack, Pat and Brack, Ben. *Moms Don't Get Sick*. Melius Publishing, Aberdeen, SD, 1990.

*A unique and wonderful book written by a mother and her young son about her breast cancer experience.*

Brady, Judy, editor. *One in Three: Women with Cancer Confront an Epidemic*. Cleis Press, 1991. P.O. Box 8933, Pittsburgh, PA 15221.

*A collection of personal research and writings of women with many kinds of cancer. A comprehensive book on the politics of women's cancer.*

Bruning, Nancy. *Coping with Chemotherapy*. Ballantine Books, New York, 1985.

*Although this is an older book, it has not, to our knowledge, been improved upon. It contains a wealth of information and advice for dealing with chemotherapy.*

Clorfene-Casten, Liane. *Breast Cancer: Poisons, Profits and Prevention*. Common Courage Press, Munroe, ME, 1996.

*Examines issues of environmental pollution and ethical responsibilities of profiteering companies that produce both carcinogenic pesticides and chemotherapy drugs.*

Colmore, Perry, and Lisa Adelsberger. *Living with Breast Cancer: 39 Women and 1 Man Speak Candidly about Surviving Breast Cancer*. Andover Townsman, Andover, MA 1997.

*A striking collection of oral histories accompanied by professional photographic portraits.*

Dackman, Linda. *Affirmations, Meditations, and Encouragements for Women Living with Breast Cancer*. Harper, San Francisco, 1991.

*This book contains selections that will comfort you at all times in your experience with breast cancer.*

Gale, Augusta, R. N. *Older Than My Mother: A Nurse's Life and Triumph over Breast Cancer*. Ananse Press, Seattle, 1996.

Goodman, Michelle. *Vanishing Cookies: Doing OK When a Parent Has Cancer*. The Benjamin Institute for Community Education and Referral. Downsview, Canada, 1990.

*A useful book for children.*

Groopman, Jerome, M.D. *The Measure of Our Days: New Beginnings at Life's End*. Penguin Putnam, New York, 1997.

*Dr. Groopman, an oncologist, shares very moving stories and experiences from his practice.*

Gross, Amy. *Women Talk About Breast Surgery: From Diagnosis to Recovery*. Clarkson Potter, New York, 1990.

*A wide-ranging set of women's experiences with surgical treatments for breast cancer.*

Harris, Linda Brown. *Breast Cancer: A Handbook*. Melpomene Institute, St. Paul, 1992. (Hard to find: Call 612-642-1951 for order information.)

*An invaluable guide to gathering information, understand-*

*ing the diagnosis, and choosing treatment. If possible, find this book early in your breast cancer experience.*

Hirshaut, Yashar, and Peter Pressman. *Breast Cancer: The Complete Guide.* Bantam Books, New York, 1992.

*A very helpful guide providing state-of-the-art information to lower your risks, maximize recovery, and help you through each step of diagnosis, surgery, treatment, and return to life after cancer.*

Kaye, Ronnie. *Spinning Straw into Gold.* Simon & Schuster, New York, 1991.

*A thoughtful, compassionate guide to emotional recovery from breast cancer.*

Kushner, Rose. *If You've Thought About Breast Cancer* (1993). Published by Rose Kushner Breast Cancer Advisory Center, P.O. Box 224, Kensington, MD 20895. (Call or write them for order information.)

*A concise gold mine of information about screening, diagnostic techniques, adjuvant therapies, breast reconstruction, and clinical trials on prevention.*

Lambert-Colomeda, Lorelei Anne. *Through the Northern Looking Glass: Breast Cancer Stories told by Northern Native Women.* National League of Nursing, New York, 1996.

Lerner, Michael. *Choices in Healing: Integrating the Best of Conventional and Complementary Approaches to Cancer.* MIT Press, Cambridge, MA, 1994.

*This excellent book offers an extensive bibliography in all areas.*

Love, Susan M., M.D. *Dr. Susan Love's Breast Book.* Addison-Wesley, Reading, MA, 1994.

*Widely available in both hardcover and paperback, this is the definitive source book about breast cancer. This is the one book which everyone will ask you if you have read. We would like to add a warning: Dr. Love writes very thoroughly about breast cancer and includes information about recurrence and mortality that may be frightening. Try to read only the sections of this book relevant to your present experience.*

McCoy, Linda Phelan. *Twenty Something and Breast Cancer: Images in Healing.* In Print Publishing, Sedona, AZ, 1996

Mayer, Musa. *Examining Myself: One Woman's Story of Breast Cancer Treatment and Recovery.* Faber & Faber, Boston and London, 1993.

*A well-written and thoughtful personal account.*

Mayer, Musa. *Holding Tight, Letting Go: Living with Metastatic Breast Cancer.* O'Reilly & Associates, Sebastopol, CA 1997.

*Honest and moving descriptions of confronting approaching death from forty people.*

Moch, Susan D. Allan Graubard, *Breast Cancer: Twenty Women's Stories: Becoming More Alive Through the Experience.* National League for Nursing, New York, 1995.

Moss, Ralph. *Cancer Therapy: The Independent Consumer's Guide to Nontoxic Treatment and Prevention*. Equinox Press, New York, 1992.

*A complete guide to complementary therapies.*

Nessim, Susan, and Judith Ellis. *Cancervive: The Challenge of Life After Cancer*. Houghton-Mifflin, Boston, 1991.

*A compassionate, practical resource for and about life after cancer. Addresses both the emotional and the practical life concerns.*

Royak-Schaler, Renee, and Beryl Lieff Benderly. *Challenging the Breast Cancer Legacy*. New York: HarperCollins, 1992.

Sherill, Marcia, and Nora Feller. *Portraits of Hope: Conquering Breast Cancer*. Wonderland Press/Smithmark Publishers, New York, 1998.

*This is a two-volume cased set that includes a book of 52 photographs with biographical statements and a hardcover blank journal.*

Spiegel, David, M.D. *Living Beyond Limits*. Random House, New York, 1993.

Stabiner, Karen. *To Dance with the Devil: The New War on Breast Cancer*. Dell Books, New York, 1997.

*This book examines the politics of the fight against breast cancer; it is an eye-opener.*

Strauss, Linda. *What About Me? A Booklet for Teenage Children of Cancer Patients*. Cancer Family Care, Cincinnati, OH, 1986.

Strauss, Linda Leopold. *Coping with a Person Who Has Cancer*. Rosen Publishing Co., New York, 1989.

*An excellent book about the many issues facing children and partners of cancer patients.*

Stumm, Diana. *Recovering from Breast Surgery: Exercises to Strengthen Your Body and Relieve Pain*. Hunter House, Alameda, CA, 1995.

Swirsky, Joan, and Barbara Balaban. *The Breast Cancer Handbook*. HarperCollins, New York, 1994.

*A practical and user-friendly guide.*

Vogel, Carole G. *Will I Get Breast Cancer? Questions and Answers for Teenage Girls*. Silver Burdett Press, Morristown, NJ, 1995.

*A straightforward yet ultimately reassuring book that takes the mystery out of breast cancer. This very helpful book addresses the concerns that daughters may have about breasts, cancer, and treatment.*

Wadler, Joyce. *My Breast*. Addison-Wesley, Reading, MA, 1992.

*It is possible—this book is funny. It is also a wise, feeling-filled, and intelligent story of one woman's cancer.*

Weiss, Marissa, M.D., and Ellen Weiss. *Living Beyond Breast Cancer: A Survivor's Guide for When Treatment Ends and the Rest of Life Begins*. Times Books, New York, 1997.

Wilson-Hashiguchi, Clo. *Stealing the Dragon's Fire: A Personal Guide and Handbook for Dealing with Breast Cancer*. Wilson Publishers, Bothell, Washington, 1995.

Wittman, Juliet. *Breast Cancer Journal: A Century of Petals.* Fulcrum Publishing, Golden, CO, 1993.

*Beautifully written reflections on the process of looking for ways to cope with and understand the experience of breast cancer.*

Yalof, Ina, ed. *Straight from the Heart: Letters of Hope and Inspiration from Survivors of Breast Cancer.* Kensington Publishers, New York, 1997.